The Art of Simpling

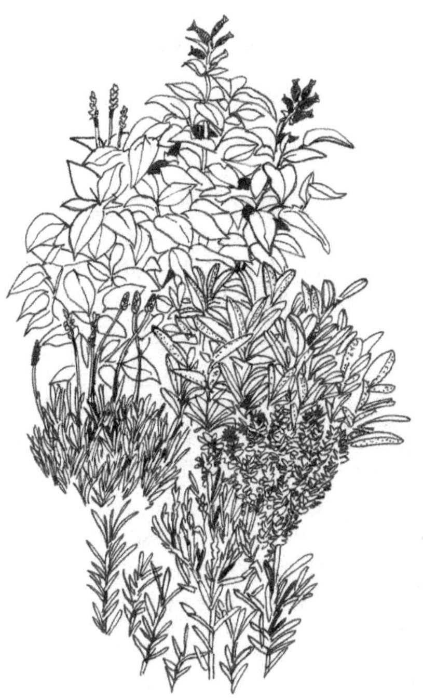

The Art of Simpling

An Introduction to the Knowledge and
Gathering of Plants

Wherein the definitions, divisions, places,
descriptions, differences, names, virtues, times
of flourishing and gathering, uses, temperatures,
signatures, and appropriations of plants are
methodically laid down.

by W. Coles

Whitworth & I • Santa Fe, New Mexico

Originally published in 1656. First Whitworth and I - Press edition, 2026.

This is a new edition of William Coles' herbal, The Art of Simpling, with updated language and spelling, as well as other copyedits, to enhance readability. The addendum to the original edition has been omitted, and excerpts from the 1657 edition have been included in chapters 1 and 25.

Original text: The Art of Simpling: An Introduction to the Knowledge and Gathering of Plants. Wherein the definitions, Divisions, Places, Descriptions, Differences, Names, Vertues, Times of flourishing and gathering, Uses, Temperatures, Signatures and Appropriations of Plants, are methodically laid down. Whereunto is added, A Discovery of the Lesser World, by W. Coles. London: J.G. for Nath: Brook at the Angell in Cornhill, 1656.

Whitworth and I - Press

Whitworth and I, LLC
223 N. Guadalupe Street, Box 283
Santa Fe, New Mexico 87501

www.whitworthandi.com

Library of Congress Control Number: on file

ISBN: 978-0-9771655-5-1

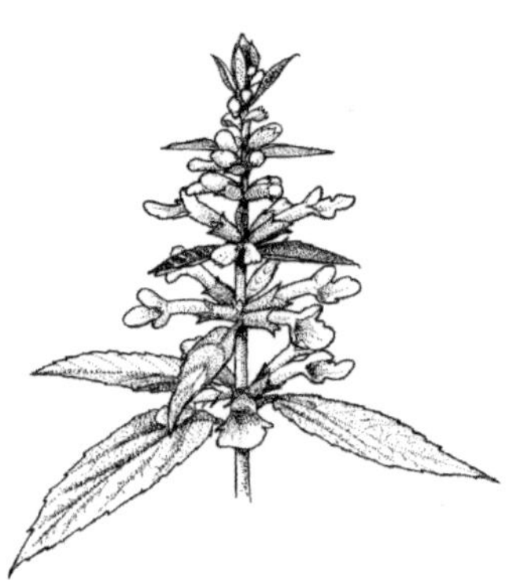

TABLE OF CONTENTS

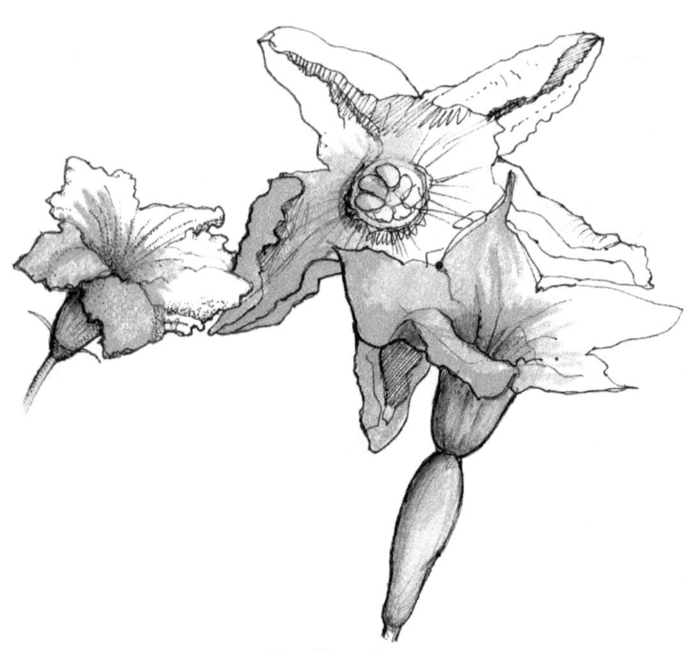

Dedication
To the most exquisite lover of plants,
Elias Ashmole, Esq.

Honoured Sir,

Though I am a stranger to your person, yet should I be so to your virtues, I might very well seem to be an inhabitant of another country, and not of this, wherein your fame is so eminent for countenancing all those that bend their endeavours to advance any kind of learning. And though I did despair the patronage of any worthy person to my well-meaning endeavours, yet since being animated by the general repute of your excellency in this kind, and the height of perfection which you have attained in this pleasant study, I do here present you with what I have expressed in the Epistle to the Reader. The result of

many years of experience, which I have employed
for the benefit of my countrymen, whose ignorance
in the forms of simples is very much to be pitied.
In commiseration whereof, I have made it my care
to muster up a number of such observations as may
tend much to their benefit, if so be they can lay aside
their self-conceitedness and diligently follow what is
here prescribed. I go not about to deceive them with a
few empty notions, as Mr. Culpeper hath lately done,
telling them many nonsensical stories of I know not
what; when as it is evident to those that knew him, or
are able to judge of his writings, that he understood
not those plants he trod upon. And that which adds to
his fallacious assertions is that he hath obtruded these
things upon the country people, persuading them
that they would be much for their benefit; who being
taken with any novelty, swallowed his bait, hoping
that there might be somewhat of value in them, but
were too much deceived, as experience may plainly
show. All the rocks at which he willingly stumbled,
I shall carefully avoid, and plainly demonstrate to
their senses the reasonableness, pleasure and profit of
what I propose. The way to make men skillful in any
art is to acquaint them thoroughly with the subject
matter thereof, as also with the principles belonging
thereunto, without which nothing but confusion
can be expected. I have therefore contrived a short
method which will accompany them in all places,
and like a mercurial statue discover unto them the
differences of plants, by the observation of which
they may make a speedy progress in the knowledge of
them to their great advantage and satisfaction.

And being assured how much you are particularly addicted to the admiration of those exquisite forms and wonderful varieties of those vegetable creatures, and of your ability to judge betwixt the fawning language of a smooth-tongued flatterer and the faithful dealing of a good commonwealth-man, I crave leave to commit it to your protection, which if you shall vouchsafe unto it, I shall not value the snarls of any self-interested persons. And thus, I humbly kiss your hands and subscribe my self.

Your very humble servant,
Will. Coles
Putney, February 22, 1655

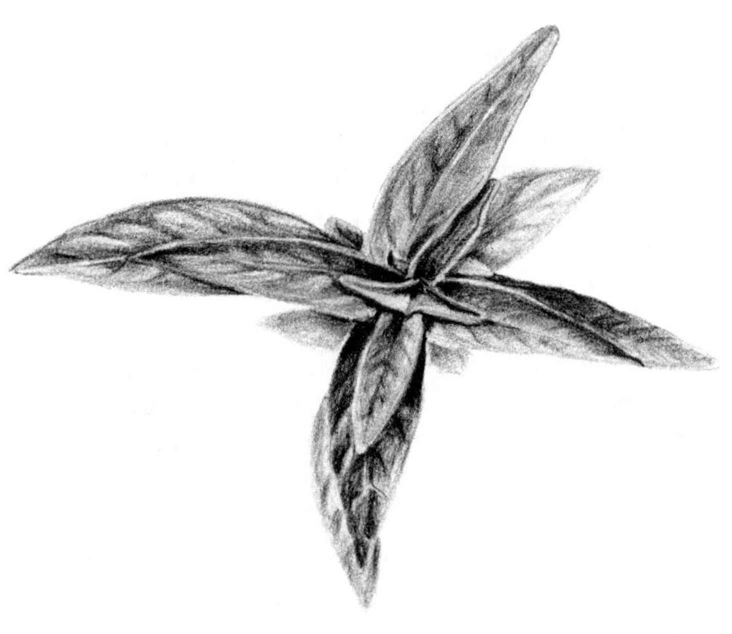

Preface

Gentle Reader,

    What a rare happiness was it for Matthioli, that famous simpler, to live in those days wherein (as he himself reports) so many emperors, kings, archdukes, cardinals, and bishops did favor his endeavors, and plentifully reward him! Whereas in our times, the art of simpling is so far from being rewarded that it is grown contemptible, and he is accounted a simple fellow who pretends to have any skill therein. Truly it is to be lamented that the men of these times, who pretend to so much light, should go the way to put out their own eyes, by trampling upon that which should preserve them, to the great discouragement of those that have any mind to bend their studies this way.

Notwithstanding, for the good of my native country, which everyone is obliged to serve upon all occasions of advantage, and in pity to such mistakers, I have painfully endeavored plainly to demonstrate the way of attaining this necessary art, and the usefulness of it, in hopes that this embryo thrown thus into the wide world, will fall into the lap of some worthy persons who will cherish it, though I knew not any to whose protection I might commend it. However, I have adventured it abroad and, to express my real affection to the public good, have in it communicated such notions as I have gathered, either from the reading of several authors, or by conferring sometimes with scholars, and sometimes with country people; to which I have added some observations of mine own, never before published, most of which I am confident are true, and if there be any that are not so, yet they are pleasant.

The result whereof will appear to the understanding reader to be this: That to be well versed in the forms and verities of plants is no such contemptible matter, as some suppose, but that God may be glorified and the Commonwealth profited as much, if not more, by this study than any whatsoever. For if every herb shows that there is a God, as verily it doth—the very beauty of plants being an argument that they are from an intellectual principle—what lectures of divinity might we receive from them, if we would but attend diligently to the inward understanding of them? And botany, being one of the handmaids to physick, and every plant being useful for somewhat or other, why should they be less respected than others, especially seeing they tend to the preservation and recovery of health, which everyone is by nature engaged to prefer before any other earthly blessing, and therefore ought principally to be respected? But physicians, and others who ought to be skilled therein, do for the most part so much affect ignorance, that they care not for having the scales thereof removed from their eyes. If they did, they should no longer continue idle but would immediately set about this ingenious exercise. Perhaps the difficulty of attaining to so intricate a knowledge might formerly be pleaded; but now that obstacle being removed out of the way, there is no excuse that I know remaining. If therefore anyone will be persuaded to entertain good thoughts of this art, he shall have here such rules as will be very helpful to him in the discovery of simples, from which he shall receive abundance of content and satisfaction. Let him make use of them, and according as he findeth, judge. If any profit redound unto him thereby, as I doubt not but there will, I shall have my desire; which is, that all sorts of learning may be promoted, but especially this despised, though advantageous art of simpling.

    I know that pieces of never so exact and curious frame, composed by the most excellent and evenest hand, cannot pass through the critical and censorious multitude without receiving the adult effects of their malignant humors so that I may not expect to escape scot-free; but if there be any one

that shall carp too much at these my endeavors, I
shall desire him to better them, if he can. Yet in hope
of a candid reception, I have hereunto annexed a
small treatise of anatomy of the parts of the body
of man, very useful for young practitioners; and as
I shall find these my first endeavors approved of by
the ingenious, I shall accordingly be encouraged
to publish the Anatomy of Plants, being a treatise
of the most known simples growing in England
and the dominions thereof, physically applied to
each particular disease; incident to each part of the
body, either of man or woman; with the easy way of
cures of the most malignant diseases, which may be
performed with a small cost, wherein every person
may be his own physician; contrived in a new and
exact method, and enriched with many observations,
not taken notice of by any other authors. The book is
well-nigh finished, and I hope will be shortly ready
for the press.

Farewell.

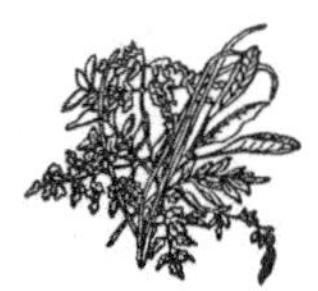

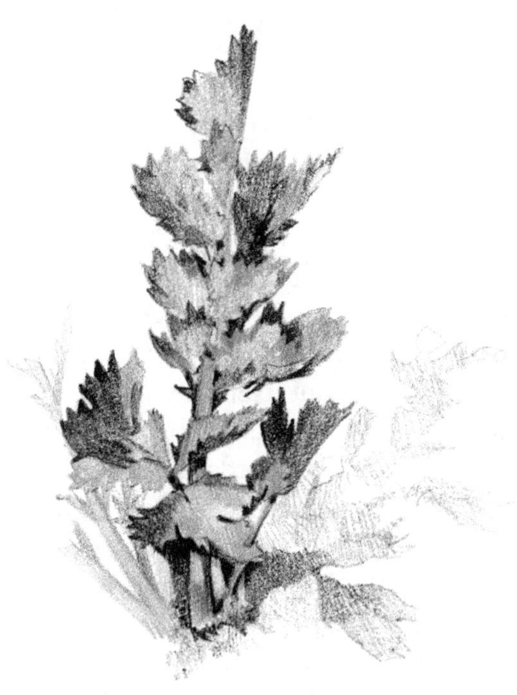

An Introduction to the Knowledge of Plants

Of Simpling, its Antiquity, Dignity, Pleasure, and Usefulness in Physick, et cetera

Simpling is an art which teaches the knowledge of all drugs and physical ingredients, but especially of plants, their divisions, definitions, differences, descriptions, places, names, times, virtues, uses, temperatures, and signatures. An art sufficiently derided by the ignorant and self-conceited but held in admiration by all those who have received any glimpse of the beauty of it. It is a subject as ancient as the Creation (as the scriptures witness), yea more ancient than the sun, or moon, or stars, they

1

being created on the fourth day, whereas plants were the third. Thus, did God even at first confute the folly of those astrologers who go about to maintain that all vegetables in their growth are enslaved to a necessary and unavoidable dependence on the influences of the stars; whereas plants were, even when planets were not. [*See footnote at the end of this chapter]

It prostitutes not itself to vulgar persons or capacities, as mechanic arts do, but is courted by emperors, kings, queens, lords, ladies and other personages of great qualities and parts. Though many physicians are too lazy now as to slight it, yet heretofore not only they, buy many noble men and women did study this part of physick, then which they desired nothing more. Nothing seemed to them more magnificent, or princely, than *scire potentates herbarum usumque medendi*. How renowned is the fame of Mithridates, King of Pontus, to this day, who indeed deserved to be remembered for his skill in twenty-two several languages? Yet he would not have been so often called to mind had he not invented that famous electuary called mithridate, which he could never have done if he had not had skill in this very art.

Medea was a king's daughter, and yet how excellently was she versed herein. The pleasure that is received from it no man knows but he that is acquainted with it. What a pleasant thing it is for a man (whom the ignorant think to be alone) to have plants speaking Greek and Latin to him, and putting him in mind of stories, which otherwise he would never think of. It will yield a man discourse wherever he goes, (travel he by sea or by land) that will render him *facundus comes*, and such a one, *in via pro vehiculo est*. With what rare colours and sweet odours do the flourishing fields and gardens entertain the senses? The usefulness of it no judicious man can deny, unless he would also deny the virtues of herbs, which experience itself doth daily approve. For how often do we see, not only men's bodies, but even the minds of those that are even distracted, to be cured by them? I know there be many physicians who hold it a disparagement to think of such small matters, and therefore they leave this office to the apothecaries, who for the most part are as ignorant as themselves and rely commonly upon the words of the silly herb-women, who many times bring them quid pro quo, then which nothing can be more sad. So, by reason of this ignorance in simples, their medicines oftentimes sort not their wished but sometimes contrary effects, to the great prejudice of their patients. Therefore, I hold it more than convenient that all those who deal in physick or surgery should be skilled not only in the qualities but also the forms of simples. For though a man knows the qualities never so well, and knows not the form, he will be at a notorious loss; but when both are rightly known and applied, they cure diseases, resist poisons, heal sores, yield food, make sauces, and whatnot, even at little or no charge.

[* *In the 1657 edition, the latter part of the first paragraph read as follows:* It is a subject as ancient as Creation, plants being a production of the third day. Notwithstanding which, I cannot readily close with their opinion who over-confidently deny the sun, moon, and stars to have any influential power upon vegetables, *et cetera,* by apprehending that plants had the precedence of Creation, because (upon a superficial view of the text) the sun seems not to have been made until the fourth day. For though that light which we now behold contracted in the sun was not drawn together into that body until the fourth day, yet was the same created before, and such its collection made up from the scattered parts of that primitive and aethereal light, which received creation upon the first day, and which until the fourth continued dispersed, darting and rowelling, through the highest part of the Creation, bestowing some proportion both of heat and influence upon those new created vegetables, though not so vigorously powerful and certain as when it was afterwards shut up within the narrower compass of that illustrious globe.]

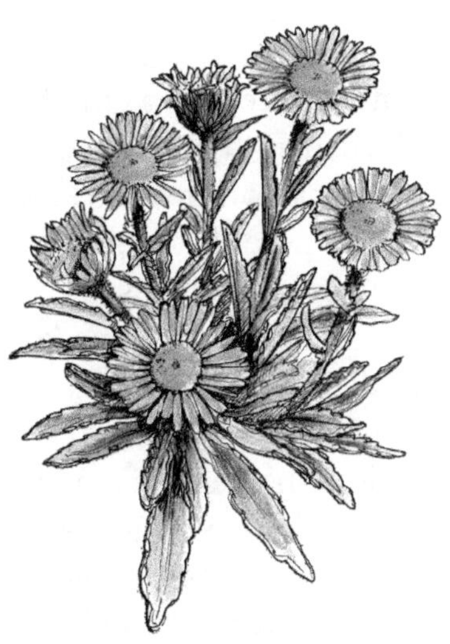

That This Art is Also Necessary for Those Who Intend to Be Divines

It is conceived under favor, that though this knowledge is especially necessary for physicians, apothecaries, chirurgeons, and such as deal in medicines; yet it would be useful to many other professions; but because divinity is the noblest of them, I will speak only to that at present.

There are in scripture several expressions and similitudes, either concerning plants or derived from them, which cannot thoroughly be understood without this art. There is mention not only of grass, herbs and trees in general, but of the tree of knowledge of good and evil and the tree of life, either of which would admit of a particular discourse, the fig tree, whose leaves our first parents sewed together to make them aprons, and of gopher wood. There is mention also of lentils, wherewith Jacob made pottage and sold them for Esau's birthright; of balm, myrrh, aloes, cassia,

frankincense, the citrine tree, the palm, the myrtle, the
willow, the vine, the cedar, the bramble, and of other
trees; of gourds, hemlock, wormwood, anise, cumin,
et cetera. Here we may note that aloes and *Lignum
aloes*, though in scripture they be used for one and the
same thing, yet they are not so, the one being the juice
of a sea-plant, the other the wood of a very beautiful
tree. It would be tedious to reckon up the materials
of the ark and of Solomon's temple, and to give the
reason why such wood, and such stones, and such
metals were used. That the lilies amongst the thorns
were woodbines is not known to everyone, or that the
husks which the prodigal son did eat were the fruit
of a tree, or that amárantos, which Saint Peter puts
for a thing that fades not away, is a flower which will
endure for a very long while.

    I could have reckoned up many more, which
for brevity sake I omitted, for understanding of the
inward meaning whereof no small skill is required.
Give me leave to give you an instance in the words
of Hosea 10:4. *"They have spoken words falsely, in
making a covenant; thus judgement springeth up like
hemlock in the furrows of the field."* For illustration of
which place, the very evil, dangerous, and poisonous
qualities of that pernicious weed would be considered,
which sometimes springs up in such places where
better grain is expected, that so it may more plainly
appear that the judgement of those magistrates the
prophet speaks of was not just, but stunk like hemlock
in the nostrils of the Almighty, and was as dangerous
to the politick welfare of the people as hemlock was
to the health of their bodies. This is mine own gloss,

how consonant to the text, or what commentators write thereon, I leave to the judgement, or at least the search of the learned divines; but for some that profess themselves to be so, I doubt whether they know what hemlock is.

If I should ask one of our upstarts what those things were which Reuben bringing home, his mother Leah and Rachel kept such a clutter about, I wonder what answer he would make? I believe he would say they were mandrakes; and if I should demand again what mandrakes were, I suppose he would say he could not tell, (an answer unbeseeming his profession) or, which is worse, that they were roots growing in proportion like a man's body, which make a wonderful shrieking at their pulling up, and perhaps that they cause fruitfulness in women, if they carry the same near their bodies. Whereas in mandrakes there is no such proportion, shrieking or vert, as every one that knows them can tell. I know not how the translators of the Bible came to mistake, but the word in the original is a common word, signifying amiable and sweet smelling flowers, (and is used, Canticles 7:13, in the same sense) which Reuben brought home for their beauty and smell, rather than their vert, whereas in the flowers of mandrake there is no such delectable or amiable smell. This is the judgement of Mr. Gerard, whose reasons for the same you may see, if you consult his herball. Those which are skilled in the original, would do well to compare the mandrake and it together with the circumstances, and see if it be not so. Thus, if a divine were a good herbarist, he might be much more accurate in the interpretation of scripture than many in our days are.

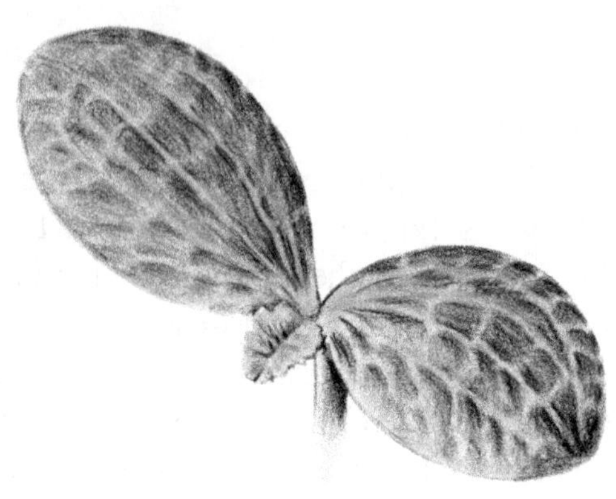

Of the Restorers of this Kind of Philosophy, of Some of the Chief Writers Thereof, and of Some Skillful Men Now Living

Though we gather from the scriptures that there was no plant whereof Adam understood not the name or virtue before his Fall; yet after that, as the world grew elder in time and so grosser in ignorance, this kind of philosophy was almost, if not altogether, forgotten. Insomuch that the Graecians, who are said to be the inventers of all arts and sciences, except the mathematics, attribute the invention hereof to Chiron the famous centaur. Doubtless Chiron was a great restorer of it, whom the poets feign to be no less than the son of Saturn and Philyra, from whom chironium, that is, centaury, takes its name. To this renowned doctor was Aesculapius the son of Apollo, set to school, who came to that perfection in physique that among the ancients he was reputed the God thereof. He was schoolmaster also to Achilles, that magnanimous Grecian captain, from whence *Achillea*, that is, milfoil, took is name.

The scripture tells us of Solomon, that he spoke (I conceive he wrote) of trees, from the Cedar which is in Lebanon to the moss that growth upon the wall, for so the best translations have it; but his books, with the writings of many others, are lost. The chiefest and ancientest that remain are those of Theophrastus, Dioscorides, Pliny, Galen, *et cetera.*, who have done rarely upon this subject, as also some later Arabians, as Avicenna, Serapion, Mesue, Rhasis, *et cetera*. Neither hath our nation been without its Gerard and Parkinson, who have bestowed much labour and travail in their voluminous herballs.

Besides these, there have been many more which have been excellently well versed in simpling, though we find not that they committed their knowledge to writing. Such as were Lysimachus King of Thrace, from whom *Lysimachia*, that is, willow-weed had its name; Gentius King of Illyria, from whom *Gentian*; Artemisia Queen of Caria, from whom *Artemisia*, that is mugwort, takes its name; Evax, Cyrus, Diocletian the emperor, *et cetera*. Those that I have known most famous in my time here in England are Doctor How, one of the masters of the physick garden at Westminster; Mr. Crosse, sometimes one of the Esquire Bedells of the University of Oxford; Master Robert Gardiner of the physick garden there; and Master Morgan the gardener at Westminster, who are most expert herein; but especially my much-honored friend, Master William Brown of Magdalen College, to whom I acknowledge myself beholden, for part of my little skill.

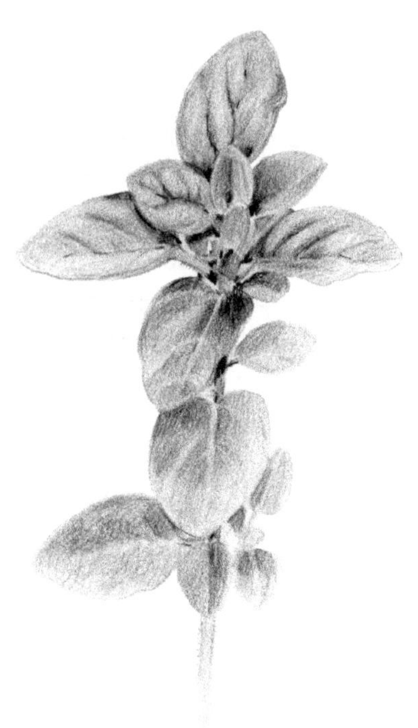

Of the Subject Matter of the Ensuing Treatise

So much for the Porch. We come now to the structure, which will not be great. The materials that we shall use in the rearing of it will be drugs, but especially plants. By drugs I mean those physical ingredients which are brought out of foreign countries such as pepper, cloves, cinnamon, myrobalan, agaric, sagapenum, sarcocolla, *Sassafras*, Lignum aloes, sealed earth, bolearmeniack, *et cetera*. But of these I shall say little more than only name, because we shall endeavor to keep our selves within the bounds of our own country, whose good it is we especially aim at.

By plants I mean whatsoever the superficies of the Earth doth put forth, if it be endued with a vegetative Soul, and that only. And of these there are five several sorts: trees, bushes, shrubs, herbs, and neuters. Trees are plants which rise out of the ground with one substantial stem, which is called the trunk or body, and afterwards spread themselves into diverse arms and branches: as oaks, pear trees, elms, ashes, *et cetera*. Bushes are those which rise out of the ground with many stalks, which afterwards put forth themselves into many lesser boughs: as roses, osiers, thorns, elder, *et cetera*. Shrubs are of a woody substance, yet do not much exceed the bigness of some herbs: as butcher's-broom, lavender cotton, ground-pine, southernwood, *et cetera*. Herbs are those whose footstalks cannot be reckoned to be wood, but do for the most part consist of leaves: as fennel, everlasting, balm, mints, *et cetera*. Neuters are those which have neither boughs nor leaves: as moss, toadstools, sponges, *et cetera*. This is the usual division of plants, which whether it be exact or not, I refer myself to the judicious reader. Of trees, bushes, shrubs and neuters, I may treat occasionally, but I shall bend my endeavors to speak especially of herbs, to whose sub-division I must proceed.

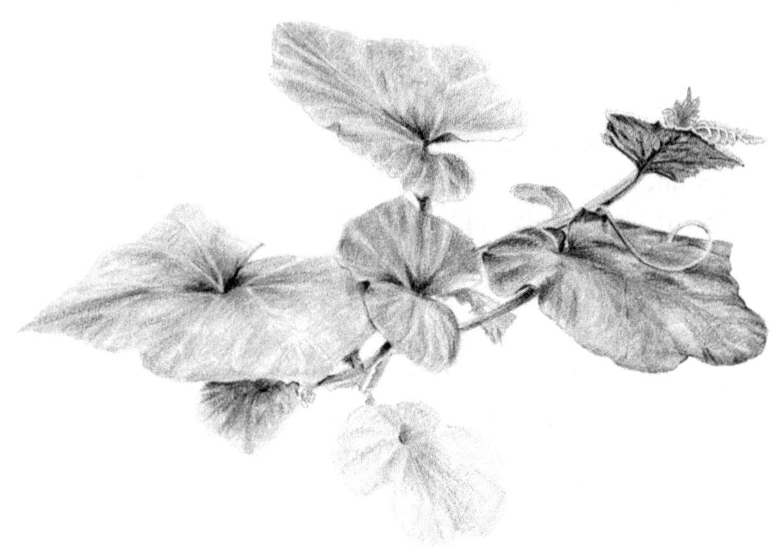

Of the Sub-Division of Herbs

As there be several divisions of plants, so there be also sub-divisions, which I shall sum up in this heptad: (1) potherbs, (2) breadcorn, (3) pulse, (4) physical herbs, (5) flowers, (6) grass, and (7) those which we in England call weeds.

By potherbs, I mean those we boil or eat raw, whether roots, fruits, or tender stalks and leaves: as turnips, carrots, radishes, leeks, onions, chives, cucumbers, melons, pompions, lettuce, parsley, sorrel, *et cetera*. By breadcorn, all sorts of wheat, rye, barley, oats, rice, panick, *et cetera*. By pulse, peas, beans, vetches, tares, lupines, *et cetera*. By physick herbs, I mean them that are so called (outstandingly so) for otherwise all are so, more or less; and those are found either in gardens, as Angelica, dragons, masterwort, Solomon's-seal, elecampane, licorice, saffron, *et cetera*, or in the fields, as tormentil, agrimony, fluellen, wood sorrel, *et cetera*. By flowers, snapdragons, lilies, iris, narcissus, larkspurs, tulips, agrimonies, hyacinths, *et cetera*. By grass, *Satyrion*, knapweed, scabious, yarrow, pearl-grass, dog-grass, trefoil, daisies, crowfoot, lady's bedstraw, *et cetera*. I find no word for a weed, either in Latin or Greek, yet because it is so common a word in England, I make that a kind, and thereof are chickweed, horehound, archangel, leavers, groundsel, nettles, hemlock, bindweed, poppy (which some call red weed), cockle, mayweed, *et cetera*.

This is a division (I confess) I never met with in any author, and some faults happily may be found in it; but herein you may perceive that I endeavor (as much as I can) to condescend to capacities of the vulgar, whose good I heartily wish.

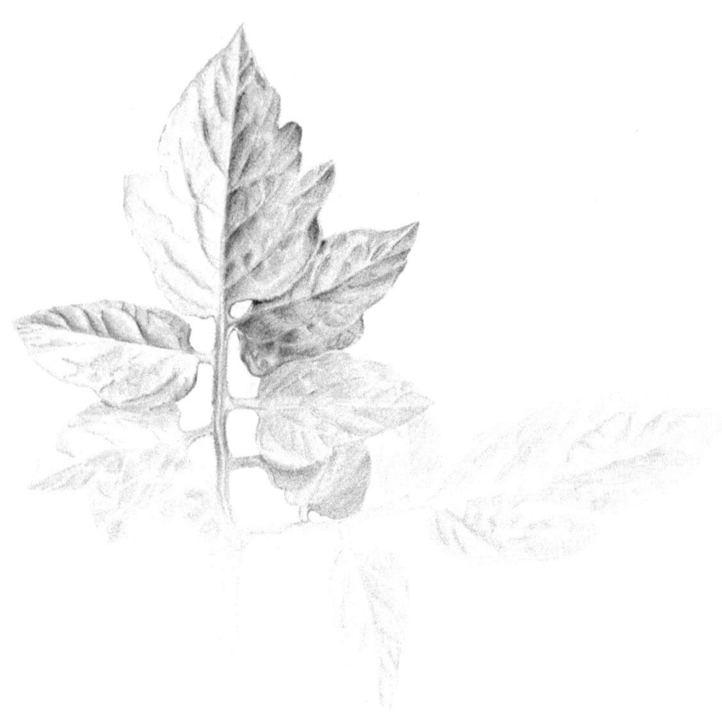

Of the Proper Places Where Plants
are to be Found

But may not some say, what tell you us of these herbs? We know not where they grow; or if you should tell us, we might as soon find them as a needle in a botte of hay; for how should we tell how to know the forms of them, or what they be like? I shall therefore first lead you to some of the places where they grow, for it would be an Herculean labour to undertake them all; and then I shall endeavor to make them known to you. Everyone I suppose knows, or may easily learn of his neighbors, what plants grow in their gardens, and therefore I will not trouble you with them.

Come into the fields then, and as you come

along the streets, cast your eyes upon the weeds, as you call them, that grow by the walls and under the hedge sides, and it will be an hundred to one if you do not find there vervain, mugwort, mercury, cinquefoil, jack-by-the-hedge, wild tansy, knotgrass, wild orache, flaxweed, houndstongue, shepherd's purse, *et cetera*.

As soon as you come into the closes, there shall have yarrow, knapweed, ragwort, scabious, dandelion, lady's bedstraw, docks, daisies, wild carrots, trefoil, earthnuts, *et cetera*. When you come amongst the corn, you shall find bluebottles, poppies, restharrow, fumitory, shepherd's needle, mayweed, cockle, corn marigold, pimpernel, cow parsnip, bindweed, sowthistles, *et cetera*.

Thence march to the woods, and there you shall have wood spurge, tormentil, agrimony, lady's mantle, St. John's-wort, wood betony, wood sorrel, satyrion, mouse-ear, moonwort, *Cistus*, milkwort, *et cetera*.

And from thence into the meadows, and there will be marsh marigolds, moneywort, meadowsweet, burnet, cockscomb, lousewort, saxifrage, meadow rhubarb, *et cetera*.

Thence to the bogs, and there you will have horsemint, cottongrass, pennygrass, butterwort, buck-beans, stinking horsetail, the small valerian, *et cetera*.

And so to the river side, and there you shall see grow upon the banks the great valerian, comfrey, sneezewort, wintercress, Clown's all-heal, the great dock, water-hemp, willow-weed, flower-de-luce, water betony, *et cetera*. Cast your eyes between the banks, and there in the water you may behold the water lily, watermilfoil, frogbit, calthrops, bur-reed, water plantain, arrowhead, water parsley, all sorts of flags, bulrushes, *et cetera*. And coming home by the ditches, you shall find duckmeat, brooklime, water-crowfoot, watercress, water parsnips, water horehound, water scorpion grass, horsemint, *et cetera*.

Coming into the town again, lift up your eyes to the walls and there you may chance to see maidenhair, wall-bugloss, whitlowgrass, polypody, rocket, wallflowers, pellitory, *et cetera*. Look a little higher toward the house tops, and you may at a distance view sengreen, or houseleek, stonecrop, herb-Robert, *et cetera*.

Now you cannot but say I have named a great many herbs, but you may perhaps say, to what purpose? Do but observe that herbs in their proper places have the greatest virtues, though happily they may be found in other places; and you find that I have wrote to much purpose. And though some may grow in diverse places, yet others are so confined, that they cannot be brought into a garden. Some of those which grow in the water, will not easily be persuaded to grow anywhere else; and so it is likewise with those which delight in dry places. You may seek some plants in some places till your eyes drop out and never find them; so true is that of the poet, *Non omnia fert omnia tellus*.

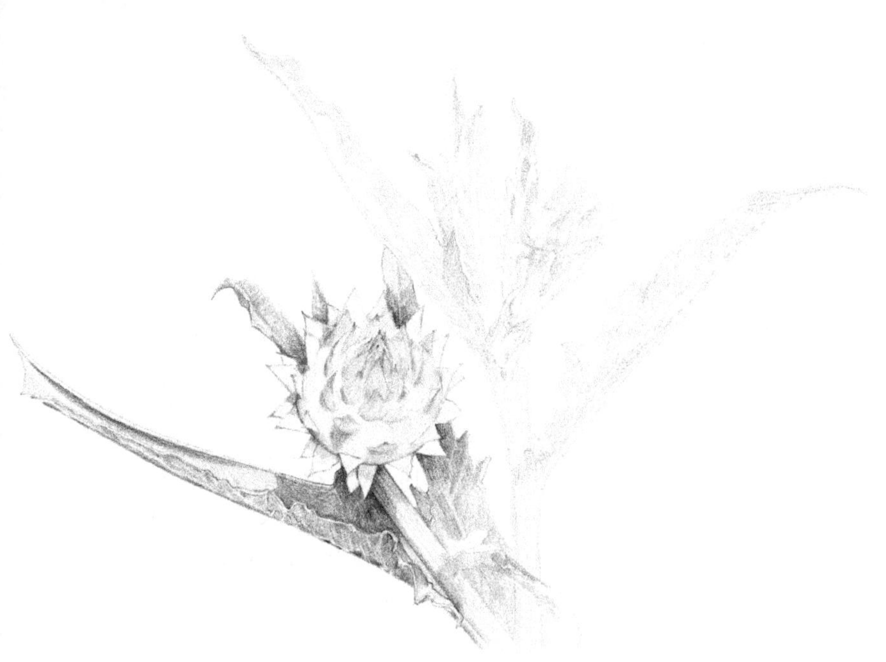

Of the Parts of Herbs

Having laid this foundation of our little edifice by acquainting you with the kinds of herbs and their places (for the trees, bushes and shrubs are bigger, and so consequently easier to be found and known), I shall proceed to the building itself, and in it give you some delineations of their parts which the exactest herberists divide into similar and dissimilar.

The similar are those five which are of one and the same substance, and cannot be divided into other arts; and because they have no proper names of their own, they do by a kind of analogy borrow them from the parts of living creatures, as: (1) flesh, (2) nerves, (3) veins, (4) skins, and (5) juice. Flesh is the more substantial part of a plant, and doth many times admit of all dimensions, as in pears, apples, plums,

melons, cucumbers, and such like fruits; the flesh is
that which is contained under the skin.

Nerves and veins are by some comprehended
under the name of fibers and are dispersed throughout
the whole plant, as nerves and veins are in living
creatures, which may easily be disjoined from the
flesh, according to their longitude. But there is a
difference betwixt them, for nerves are smaller and
dryer, but the veins are greater and, being hollow,
do contain in them that moisture which gives
nourishment to the plants. That hollowness, though it
cannot easily be seen, yet it may be perceived by the
juice they send forth, which is sometimes white, as in
spurge, sowthistles, *et cetera*, and. sometimes yellow,
as in celandine.

The skin is that wherewith the stalks, boughs,
leaves, fruits, and sometimes the roots are covered,
as with a thin garment. The juice (which in this place
doth comprehend also the tear) is answerable to
the blood in living creatures; but the juice squeezes
out after pounding, the tear dropping out of its own
accord.

The dissimilar parts are those wherein the
similar parts are contained, which are likewise five:
(1) roots, (2) stalks, (3) leaves, (4) flowers, and (5)
seeds. The root is the lowermost part of a plant, which
answers to the mouth in a man and, being fastened in
the earth, draws convenient nourishment unto it, and
supplieth all its parts.

The stalk is that part of a plant which riseth
up from the root, and is as it were a pipe to convey
the nourishment, being more fully concocted to the

rest of the parts, within which many times there is the pith, which consists of flesh, and sometimes of fleshy nerves and moisture.

The leaf is that part of a plant which is sent forth from the main stalks by another lesser stalk and consists of three similar parts, to wit: veins, sinews, and flesh.

The flower is the beauty of the plant, arising from the most refined and concoctedest matter, and therefore is most commonly of a different colour from the leaves, as yellow, blue, red, white, and sometimes mixed.

The seed is that part of the plant which is ended with a vital faculty to bring forth its like, and it contains potentially the whole plant in it.

These are the best definitions I could find or invent, which I did the rather set down, because I shall have occasion to treat of the differences which arise from them, but especially from the roots, stalks, leaves, flowers and seeds, in some of which we shall now and then occasionally show you certain diagnostics, or tokens, whereby you may be infallibly informed how to distinguish one herb from another.

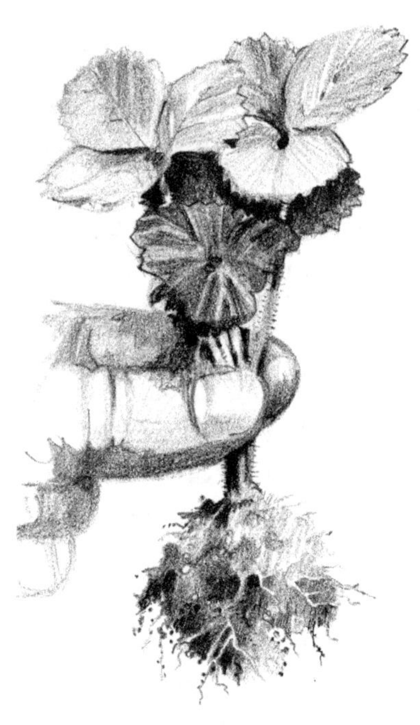

Of the Differences of Roots

Herbs differ much in their roots, whereof the figures of some are long, some round, some straight, some crooked, some shallow, some deep, some bulbous, some like to external forms, some soft, some hard, some hollow, some knotty, *et cetera*. Those that are long are parsnips, carrots, radishes, and bryony. The round are turnips, potatoes, and onions. Some are straight, as garden cresses, orache, wormseed, and mustard. Some are crooked, as rocket, spurge, and bluebottle. Those whose roots are but shallow are chickweed, moss, liverwort, and stonecrop. Those that go deep into the earth are elecampane, horseradish, and sorrel, whose root goeth farthest into the earth of any herb, insomuch that it hath been known to go three cubits deep, as my Lord Bacon witnessed in his *Historia Naturalis*. You shall see some bulbous, as tulips, daffodils, garlic, saffron, and hyacinths. Some are like to external forms, as the roots of asphodel to an acorn, of palma Christi to a hand, of other, satyrions to dogstones, goatstones, *et cetera*.

It is said by some that the roots of Solomon's-seal, are like a seal, and therefore so called; but I think rather with Master Gerard, that it is from the wonderful faculty it hath in sealing up burstnesses and green wounds. You shall have some roots hard, as the greater centaury, gromwell, parsley and mallows, and some soft, as cabbage, Alexanders, skirrets and *Tragopogon*. Some are hollow, as Radix cava, that is hollowroot. Others are knotty, as the roots of flower-de-luce, peony, *Eryngium*, *et cetera*. Some plants there are, but rare, that have a mossy, or downy root; and likewise, that have a number of threads like beards, as mandrakes, whereof witches and imposters make an ugly image, giving it the form of the face at the top of the root, and leave those strings to make a broad beard down to the feet. Also, there is a kind of nard in Crete (being a kind of phu) that hath a hairy root, like a rough-footed dove's foot. And there is one herb flat at the bottom, and seemeth as if the nether part of its root were bit off, and is called Devil's bit, whereof it is reported that the Devil, knowing that that part of the root would cure all diseases, out of his inveterate malice to mankind, bites it off. Henbane and hemlock have roots so like a parsnip that they have been mistaken for it, to the endangering of the lives of some.

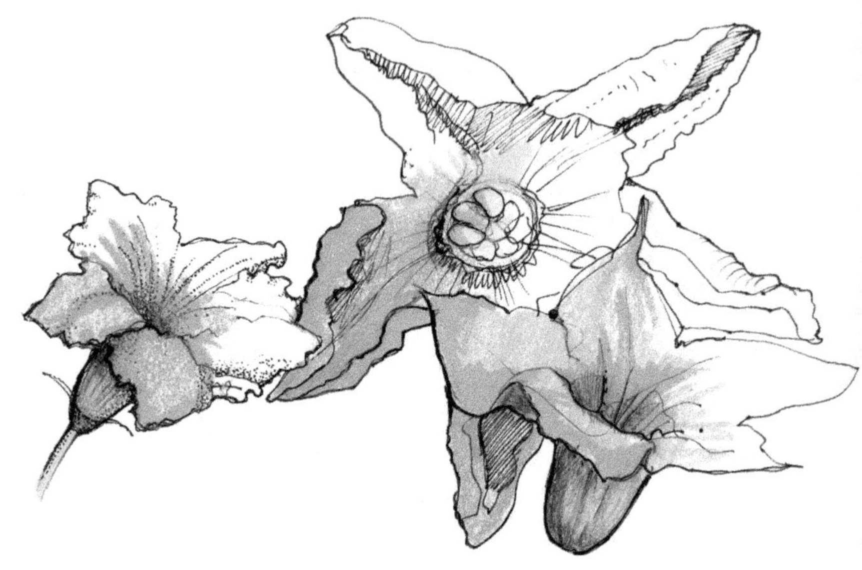

Of the Differences of Stalks

Some differences are taken also from the stalks. All chickweeds, (for there be many sorts of them) if the stalks be gently broken, you shall have in the middle of them a kind of sinew, by which you may know them from almost any plants that grow. Stalks are of diverse figures, also. Some have straight stalks, as beans, hemp, flax, and nettles; some are bending, as Solomon's-seal, snapdragon, mugwort, mercury, archangel, *et cetera*. Others lie on the ground, as peas, chickweed, pennyroyal, and pinks. Some stand bolt upright, as throatwort, Clown's all-heal, ploughman's spikenard; others spread into many branches, as vervain, larkspur, smallage, and mustard; other stalks have no branches, as woodruff, satyrion, and naked horsetail. And there be that wind one within another, as periwinkle, bindweed, and tares. Many of them have round stalks, as parsley, hemlock, and tulips; but some have angles or edges as the daffodil, which hath two, cyperus grass three; horehound, goose grass, *et cetera* are four square. Some, as orache, beets, rhubarb, coleworts, *et cetera* have red stalks, and some are white, and green. Some stalks are pecked, as dragons, scorpion grass, *et cetera*. Moth mullein and rose campion are downy; some have joints and knuckles, as clove gillyflowers, pinks, soapwort, fennel, corn, reeds and canes. The stalks of the four last being dry are hollow. Some stalks are full of milk, as lettuce, rampions, sowthistle, spurge, *et cetera*. Some have a viscous matter adhering to it, as catchfly, by which you distinguish it from the valerian that is so like it.

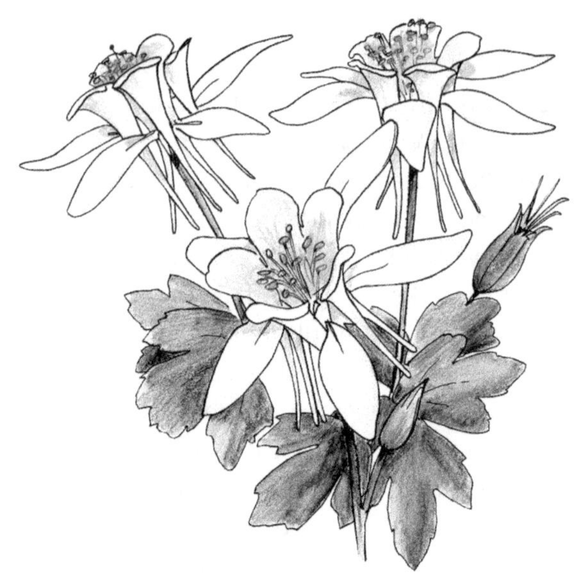

Of the Differences of Leaves

But of all the parts of herbs, the leaves afford us the greatest variety of differences. Yea they are so many, that it would puzzle a good head to find terms to express them by. As many as are obvious I shall set down, and tell you that the reason of the names of some herbs arise from their leaves.

Arrowhead is so called because the leaf of it is like the head of a barbed arrow. Scurvygrass is called spoonwort because the leaves of it represent the fashion of a spoon. Plantain is called ribwort because every leaf hath five strings somewhat like ribs. The sword flag is so called for that the leaves so nearly resemble a sword, crow foot the foot of a crow. The leaves of teasel inclosing the stalk are concavus, which receive the falling rain and retain it there, and is therefore called Venus' basin. *Tragopogon* groweth

like a goat's beard, and is therefore so named.
Twayblade is so termed for that is hath but two
leaves; trefoil for that it hath three; herb Paris hath
four; cinquefoil five; heptaphyllon seven.

The leaves of butterwort feel as if melted
butter had been powered upon the leaves. *Ros solis*,
or sundew, hath a dew upon the leaves at noon, even
in the hottest weather; shepherds call it the red rot
because it rotteth sheep. Some leaves have sand about
them always, as mercury and orache. The leaves of
all sorts of *Scabiosa* break with small strings like
hairs in the middle, by which you may know it from
knapweed, which is otherwise very like it. Saw-wort
is so called for that the leaves are nicked like a saw.
The leaves of pimpernel are speckled underneath. If
you hold the leaves of St. John's-wort and St. Peter's-
wort against the light you shall find them perforated
with holes like a sieve, the first more, the second
less. Butterbur was so called because the country
housewives were wont to wrap their butter in the
large leaves thereof.

The leaves of rhubarb, cabbage, burdock, *et
cetera* are also very large and roundish. Other docks,
tobacco, elecampane, *et cetera* have leaves long and
large, but few. Leadwort hath leaves of the colour of
lead. Thyme, rue, asparagus, spignel, fennel, *et cetera*
hath many small leaves. Those of orpine, aloes, and
houseleek are thick and oily. Stone crop hath leaves
long and round, almost as rosemary. Some are more
indented, as radish, vervain and dandelion; some less,
as maudlin, allheal, tansy, and sneezewort. Arum is
smooth and spotted; arsesmart rough and spotted, and

of this there be two sorts, biting and not biting, which
may be discerned if you lay a leaf over your tongue
and break it. Some are only rough, as comfrey, teasel,
et cetera. Bugloss is so called because it is rough like
an ox tongue. Some are smooth and glib, as bear's
breech, called branc-ursine, mandrake, *et cetera*.
Many more differences I might add, but enough is as
good as a feast.

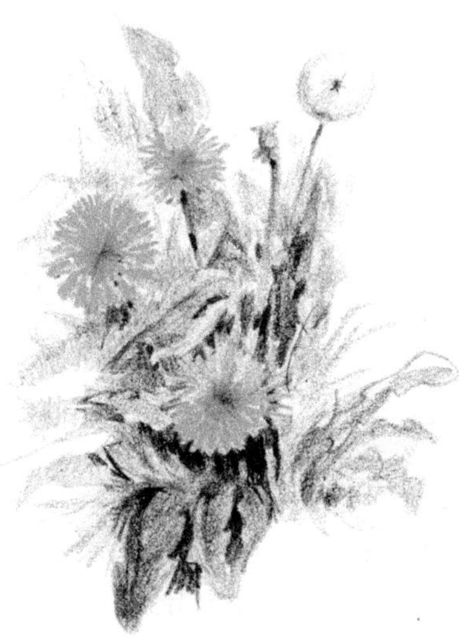

Of the Differences of Flowers, According to Their Times as Well as Figures

Neither are flowers without very many great differences, some may be taken from the times of the year wherein they flower, as the winter wolf's-bane is called Christmas flower because it puts forth its blossoms about that time, and so doth the true black hellebore. After these (and sometimes before it if the winter be mild) come primroses, crocuses, anemones, and hepaticas. The mezereon tree blossoms early too, and so do impatient lady's smocks. In February you shall have violets, daffodils, wallflowers, hyacinths, scurvygrass, chickweed, red archangel, *et cetera*.

After March come cowslips, daisies, tulips, star-of-Bethlehem, *et cetera*. April brings flower-de-luce, woodbine, cinnamon rose, *et cetera*. May brings roses, pinks, and Whitsun gillyflowers, and then dropwort, shepherd's-needle, *et cetera* do flower. In

June meadowsweet, burnet, lovage, spignel, larkspur, *et cetera*. In July come clove gillyflowers, or as some will have them July flowers, holy oaks, *et cetera*. In August, Clown's all-heal, winter cherry, *et cetera*.

In September and afterwards if the latter spring be not hindered with cold weather, strawberries, primroses, and those that flower first, will flower again.

Flowers have all exquisite figures; stock gillyflowers have seldom more than four leaves, and it is reported that they will sometimes have five, and that the seeds of them being sown will prove double, and therefore some tie a thread about them that they may know how to preserve them for seed. Those which have five are larkspurs, pinks, primroses, borage, bugloss, *et cetera*. Some have six, as the flower-de-luce, white lilies, *et cetera*. Those tulips and anemones, are (by some) reckoned to be best which have most leaves. Some put forth a great multitude of leaves, as marigolds, trefoil, *et cetera*. We see also that the sockets and supporters of flowers are figured, as in the five brethren of the rose, whereof there is this common riddle:

> Five Brethren, all in one,
> Three have beards, and two have none.

But to come to those that resemble the parts of living creatures. The flower of snapdragon, and that of wild flax, which I take to be of the same kind, is like the mouth of a lion, or rather like the snout of a calf. The flower of the dead-nettle is like a weasel's face and is called galeopsis, which in Greek signifies the same. Larkspur hath a flower with an heel like a lark. The flowers of peas, vetches, *et cetera* are somewhat like a butterfly, and there is a satyrion which represents it very much. There is another satyrion like a bee, another like a wasp. Some flowers, as the flower of the sun, marigolds, wartwort, and mallowflowers bow and incline themselves towards the sun, which happeneth because that the part against which the sun beateth, waxeth more faint and flaccid in the stalk. Others open their leaves when the sun shineth, and again in some part, close them either towards night or when the sun is overcast, as marigolds, tulips, pimpernel, *et cetera*. But goat's beard, contrary to these, is shut at noon when the sun shineth and is therefore called go-to-bed-at-noon. Some represent bells, some helmets, some fingerstalls, as foxgloves. Some boxes out of which dice are cast, as *Fritillaria*.

There be also differences of flowers of the same kind, proceeding from the colour, some white, some red, some yellow, some blue, some mixed, but especially in tulips, of which there is the white and yellow 'Crown', the 'Fool's Coat', the 'Switzer', the 'Prince', the 'Mourning Widow', *et cetera*. There be anemones, gillyflowers, *et cetera* of several colours. Some flowers grow double, as daisies, larkspur, bachelor's buttons, crowfoot, *et cetera*. Coltsfoot flowers before it putteth forth its leaves; and there is a sort of willow-weed, which hath its flowers upon the husk wherein the seed is contained, and is called in Latin *Filius ante Patrem*, that is, the father before the son, because it is more usual for an herb to flower before it seed, but in this it is otherwise.

I might be larger, but I fear I have exceeded already.

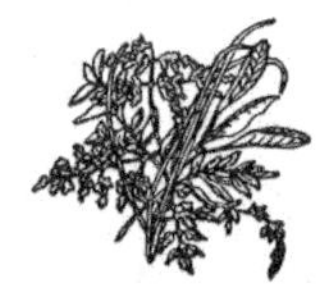

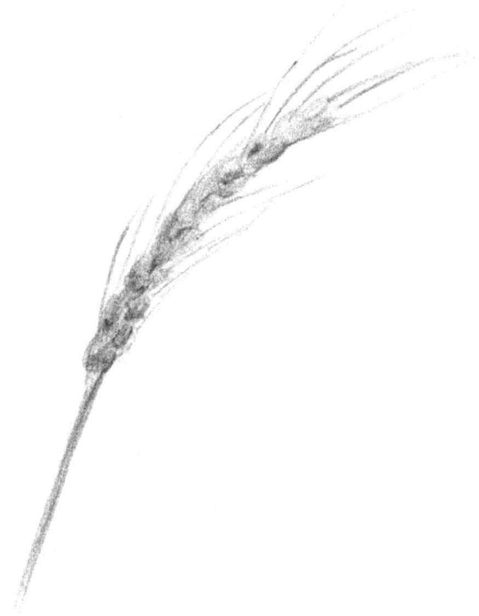

Of the Differences of Seeds

Seeds have also their differences. The seeds of all pulse grow in cods, and have several forms, whereof one hath seeds like a kidney and is therefore called the kidney bean. Other seeds grow in husks, as oats. Some grow in ears, as panick, wheat, rye, barley, *et cetera*. Lavender, and also plantain, is spiked; but the seeds of fennel, parsnip, parsley, chervil, hemlock, carrot, *et cetera* grow upon umbels of tufts.

The seed of bulronaek resembles the moon, which is therefore called great moonwort, and this seed is contained in a husk like unto white satin, which is the name of it, though our women call it honesty. The herb cranesbill is so called because the seeds are like a crane's bill; shepherd's-purse is so called, because the seeds of it resemble the leather bag wherein shepherds put their victuals. Shepherd's-needle hath seeds like needles.

Some grow in knaps like bottles, as knapweed, which some call darbottle, bluebottle, great centaury, *et cetera*. Some in berries, as those of tusan. Gromwell hath a seed as hard as a stone, and for that reason the Greeks call it *Lithospermum*. Some seeds are very rough and will stick to the garments of those that pass by, as those of burdock, agrimony, houndstongue, cleavers. Some have a kind of down fastened to them, which the wind bloweth away together with the seed, as coltsfoot, dandelion, and some thistles. If the down flyeth off when there is no wind, it is a sign of rain. Some seeds are comprehended within the flesh of fruits, as cucumbers, melons, pompions, *et cetera*.

The colours of seeds are commonly white, reddish, or black. Most seeds in the growing leave their husks or rind about the root; but the onion will carry it up, so that it will be like a Cap upon the top of the young onion. There is a plant called *noli me tangere*, near which if you put your hand, the seed will spurt forth suddenly, in so much that the unexpectedness of it made the valiant Lord Fairfax to start, as Master Robert at the physick garden in Oxford can tell you. The seeds of cotton are encompassed about with white wool; they are in shape like the tyrdels or dung of a coney.

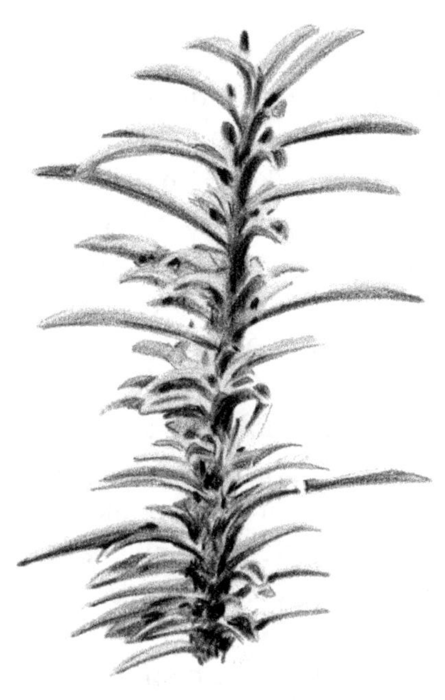

Of the Excrescences of Plants

Besides these common parts of plants, there be some excrescences that are more proper and restrained to a few, and these do commonly belong to trees and bushes, which I have made little mention of because they are more obvious. But for as much as these which I shall speak of are less known, I have thought fit to put them down in this place. There is a kind of sponge of a dusky brown colour, commonly called Judas's ear, growing at the roots of trees, but especially on the elder, on which tree some think Judas hanged himself, and therefore this sponge in Latin is called *auricula-judae*. It hath a strange property, for being put into warm water, it swelleth and openeth extremely, and is useful for

curing squinances, and inflammations of the throat.
Agaric also is a kind of spongy excrescence growing
upon the tops of oaks and other trees in the nature of
a mushroom, though it be affirmed by some that it
growth also at the roots. It is famous in physick for
purging of tough phlegm and for opening the liver,
but it is offensive to the stomach; you may have it at
the apothecary's.

Another thing which hath a strange kind of
growth is mistletoe, which is found to put forth,
not only upon, but sometimes also underneath the
boughs of crabtrees, apple trees, and hazels; the
rarest groweth upon the oaks and is counted very
medicinal, as also the polypody. I believe the thing
itself is better known than the manner of its growing,
because it is carried many miles to set up in houses
about Christmas time, when it is adorned with a white
glistering berry.

A man may count the prickles of plants to
be a kind of excrescence, for they will never be
boughs, nor bear leaves. Some have prickles upon
their boughs, and those are black and white thorns,
briar rose, rasp trees, crabtree, gooseberry, barberry,
et cetera. Others have prickles upon their leaves, as
holly, juniper, furze, thistles. Nettles and borage also
have prickles, the one venomous, the other harmless.
Another kind of excrescence is an exudation of plants
joined with putrefaction, as we see in things like
apples, which are chiefly found upon the leaves of
oaks, and sometimes upon willows. There is a kind
of prediction amongst country people that if the oak
apple broken be full of worms (as sometimes it is)

it is a sign of a pestilent year, which is probable,
because they grow of corruptions.

Of all trees, none doth bear more excrescences
than the oak, for besides the mistletoe, polypody,
oak apples, and acorns, which are the natural fruit, it
beareth galls and oak nuts, which are inflammable,
and certain oak berries, which stick to the tree without
stalk. There is also upon the wild briar a mossy
tuft of diverse colours, very easy to be seen in the
winter when the leaves are off, which if you cut in
sunder, you shall find them full of little white worms,
which in the summertime are changed into the fly
'Cantharides'. The birch tree, the nut, the walnut, and
the plane trees have on them things called in Greek
cachrys, in English catkins, or cat's tails, if I mistake
not, which are there the most part of winter. They are
of a burning quality in physick. There is a Moss the
perfumers have, which cometh out of apple trees of
an excellent sent.

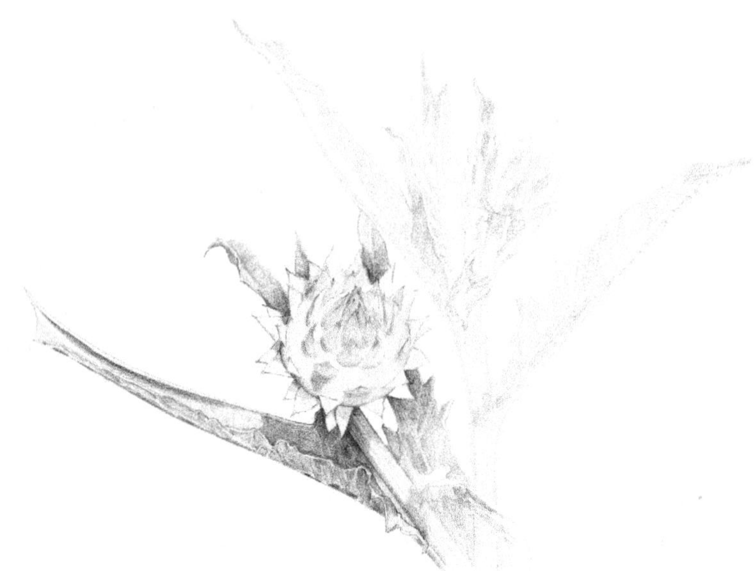

Of Smells and Tastes in Plants and Their Differences

And because there be some differences in plants, which arise from the smells and tastes, I shall take the pains to present you with some of them. There is a tree called arborvitae, or Tree of Life, whose leaves being squeezed between one's fingers, smell like unto bread and cheese. The smell of burnet is like to that of a cucumber. Stinking orange smells like old ling, and somewhat else. The smell of cresswort is like unto honey, but somewhat faint. There is a kind of willow-weed, and that very common, which smells like coddled apples. The pasque flower, called in Latin *Pulsatilla*, will bite you by the nose if you rub it between your fingers and smell to it, and so will gentian or felwort.

The leaves of coriander do smell very strong, and so do those of smallage, wormwood, rue, hemlock, henbane, *et cetera*. Sweet maudlin, marjoram, muscovy, *et cetera* are known by their sweet smells. You can scarce distinguish between chamomile and young mayweed but by the smell. The root of the little valerian is sweet like unto musk. It is reported that sweet moss, besides that upon the apple trees, groweth likewise sometimes upon the poplar.

So much for the smells, I come now to the tastes. *Spatula foetida*, or stinking Gladwin, hath a taste like unto roast beef. The stalk of the great water dock tastes like green sauce and is also as pleasant to eat as the best sorrel. Earthnuts, or as some call them pignuts, taste somewhat like other nuts. The leaves of the vine and barberry bush taste like sorrel. Rocket tastes like milk that is burnt too. Arum, or cuckoo-pint, is of a very biting taste, and so is spearwort, or water crowfoot, biting arsesmart, *et cetera*. Some plants smell little but taste very bitter, as aloes, lavender, cotton, the lesser centaury, *et cetera*. Some have a biting taste, but somewhat pleasant, as cresses, garden ginger, tarragon, *et cetera*. Seaweed, samphire, scurygrass, *et cetera* do participate of saltiness. There be fruits that are sweet before they are ripe, as myrobalans; so too are fennel seeds sweet before they ripen, and afterwards grow spicy. And some never ripen to be sweet, as tamarinds, lemons, barberries, crabs, sloes, *et cetera*. Some are very acrimonious, as euphorbia, celandine, sowthistles, spurge, old lettuce, figs from the tree, *et cetera*. There is a kind of wormwood so like lavender that it cannot be known from it but by the smell and taste.

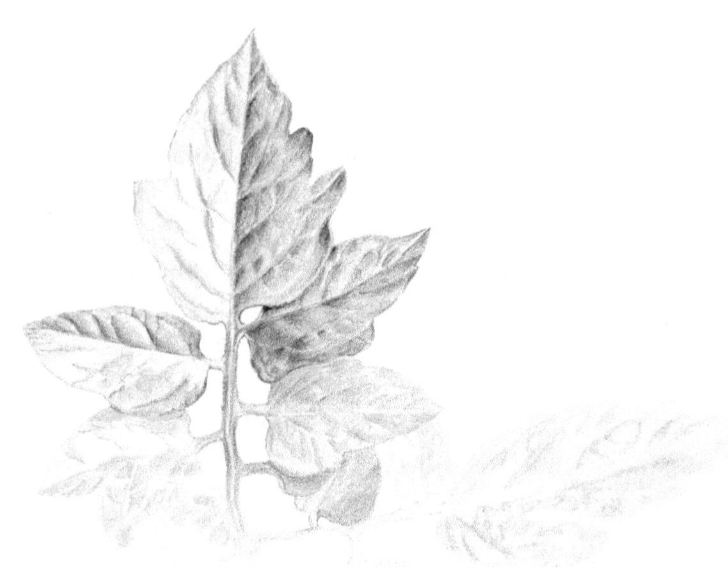

Of the Juices of Plants

Neither will it be amiss now we are speaking of the diagnostics of plants, to say somewhat more particularly of the juices also, from whence the knowledge of some of them is derived. Though the colour of most of them be green, or of a waterish colour, yet some of them are of other colours also; as the juices of figs, old lettuce, sowthistle, spurge, *et cetera* are as white as milk and are commonly so called. And here we may observe the difference between spurge and wild flax, which are somewhat alike, but that hath milk, the other none, according to the rhyming verse,

Esula lacte scit sine lacte Linaria crescit.

Euphorbia hath a kind of milk too, though not very white; and celandine hath a yellow milk, which will issue forth if it be but broken. There is hardly found a plant that yieldeth a red juice, either in the blade or ear, except it be the tree that beareth *sanguis draconis*, which groweth chiefly in the Island of Socotra, after the form of a sugar-loaf. It is likely that the sap of that plant doth concoct in the body of the tree, for we see that grapes and pomegranates are red in the juice but green in the tear; the herb *Amaranthus* (indeed) is red all over, and basil is red in the wood, and so is red sanders, but the juice of neither of them is so. The juices of flowers are commonly of the same colour with the flowers which are of a more refined and concocted matter than the stalks, yet the juices of fruits are not always so for there be black plum and red apples, neither of which have a black or red juice.

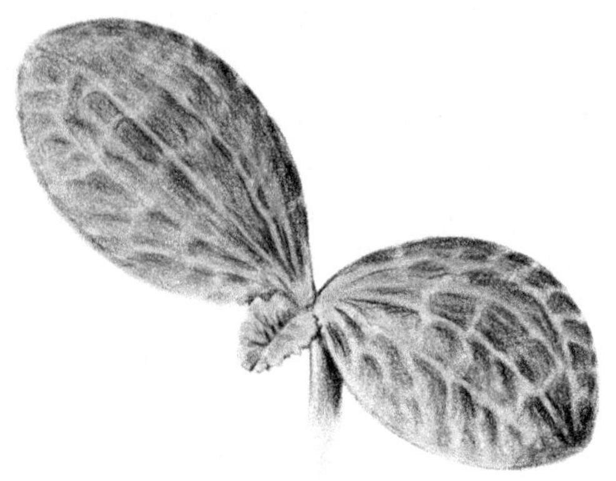

Of the Use of Plants, and First of Those Which are Alimental

The uses of plants, are reckoned up, would swell into a volume; but I shall endeavor to reduce them to as few heads as I can and begin first with those that are alimental. And here I shall not sum up those that are commonly used for aliment, as turnips, carrots, cabbage, *et cetera* but those which are less known, yea such as country people will scarce venture to eat: the tops of hops and turnips running up to seed, boiled and buttered, do eat like asparagus; the buds of broom being pickled are of an excellent relish; the roots of tulips boiled and buttered make a rare dish.

There be several ways of dressing mushrooms to make them edible; the leaves and stalks of Alexanders, being boiled, are eaten alone or with fish to correct them; the stalks are preserved raw in pickle, and presented to the table for a curious sallet. The root of *Arum* being raw, is exceeding biting, but being boiled it is good food; the roots of *Tragopogon*, or goatsbeard, boiled and buttered, as parsnips and carrots, are far better: Ashweed, which some call jump-about, boiled with bacon when it is young, is a timely dish, and so is young comfrey. Lamb's lettuce, or corn sallet, is the earliest thing that I know eaten raw. Pennyroyal chopped and put into a bag-pudding giveth it a savory relish. Good women use the buds of elders, nettle tops, watercress and Alexanders to make pottage in the springtime. Horseradish root sliced thin with a little vinegar is a wholesome sauce with mutton, and so are the leaves of Jack-by-the-hedge, which therefore by some called sauce alone.

And if you will have any more, you must go to the cooks, who can make many more dishes out of them. Yea, they can make good broth with the leg of a joynstoole, if you allow them cost. But even some of those herbs which are not esculent, are notwithstanding peculent, as hops, broom, angelica, balm, *et cetera*, which give a dainty relish to liquor if they be boiled therein. For distilled waters, you may have aniseed, mint, angelica, *et cetera*. Though plants are not now reckoned of so good nourishment as flesh, yet the Pythagorean philosophers lived longer than any in these days do.

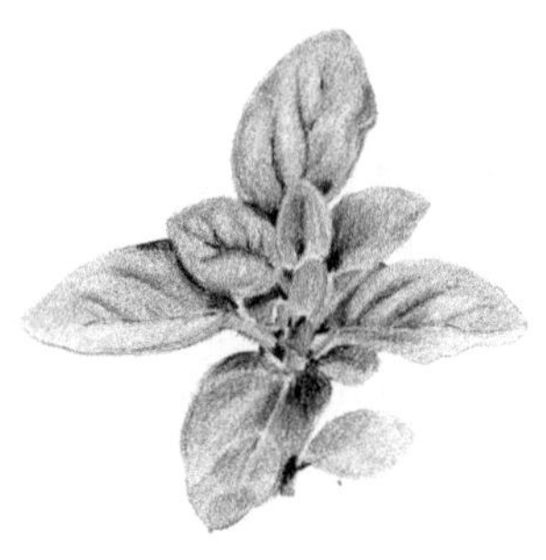

Of the Physical Use of Plants

Hence I might enter upon a plentiful harvest, but I shall only glean out some of the chiefest simples that England affords, adjoining some of their verities.

Licorice and saffron are two things, whereof without dispute our English are the best. Licorice boiled in fair water, with maidenhair and figs, maketh a very good diet drink for those which are troubled with a dry cough, or any grief of the breast and lungs. Saffron strengthens the heart exceedingly, quicketh the brain, helps consumptions of the lungs, difficulty of breathing, and is good to make stays to put to the throats of them that have the smallpox.

And as I take it, the best elecampane grows in England, the roots of which being candied with sugar, helps the cough, shortness of breath, and wheezing in the lungs. Many other plants that grow here also, are as good as the transmarine, though the druggists extoll the outlandish that they may gain thereby the more. Our rhubarb is nothing inferior to that which comes out of China, and in process of time will be as famous. It purgeth the body of choler and phlegm, and put amongst other ingredients, cleanest the stomach, liver, and blood. Our angelica is as good as that of Norway and Ireland. It is very sovereign against poison and the plague, and so is the water of the herb dragons. Our gentian is as good as that which is brought from beyond the sea, though perhaps it growth more plentifully in Italy and other places.

But England is before all the countries famous for its plenty of saxifrage. We have maidenhair here also, never a whit inferior to the Assyrian. Other physical herbs are asarabacca, which purgeth upwards and downwards. Scordium, of which diascordium is made and given to strengthen the heart and stomach, which it doth exceedingly. Wood-sorrel cools the blood, helps ulcers in the mouth, hot defluxions upon the lungs, *et cetera*. Marshmallows ease the pain of the stone. Pimpernel draws thorns and splinters out of the flesh. Smallage provokes the termes, and is singular good against the yellow jaundice. Ceterach helps the strangury, and so doth dropwort. Dwarf elder, inwardly taken, is a singular purge for the dropsy and gout. Fennel increaseth milk in nurses. Fumitory boiled in white wine and taken inwardly, helps such as are itchy and scabbed. Doe's foot helps the whine colic; periwinkle cures the cramp; plantain leaves are excellent for green wounds, the roots for the headache. Peony roots and seeds are good against the convulsion and falling sickness; shepherd's-purse stoppeth blood; houseleek is good against the shingles. The lesser centaury, wormwood, garlic, lavender cotton, and all plants that have a bitter juice kill the worms.

Let thus much suffice in brief concerning the internal, or physical, use of plants.

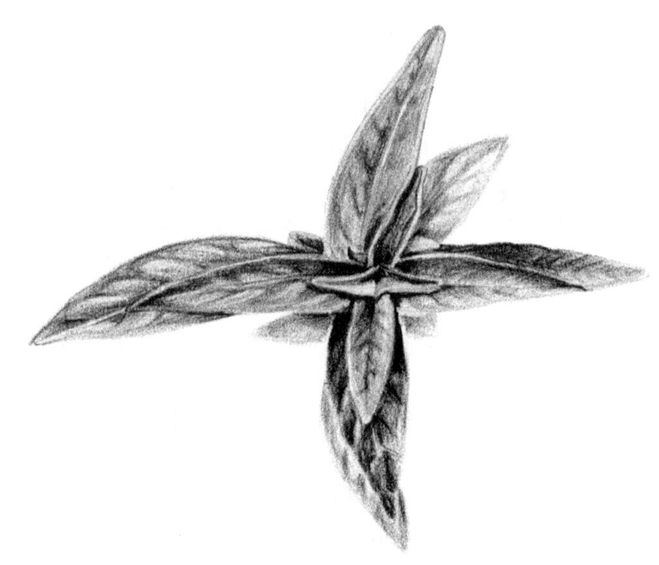

Of the Chirurgical Use of Plants

Considering how subject the body of man is to be wounded and troubled with several maladies, as felons, whitlows, itch, scabs, *et cetera*, and because there is less prejudice in applying things outwardly than inwardly, I shall here insist upon the virtues of some herbs that are useful upon this account and encourage those who are in no great danger to use them. But in dangerous cases, if a good chirurgeon be to be had, commit thyself to his daily experience rather than be penny wise and pound foolish. A sheep many time perisheth for want of a half penny worth of tare, and one spark sometimes sets a town on fire, therefore neglect not the smallest wounds, but apply some of these easy remedies which follow.

The juice or water of flaxweed put into foul ulcers, whether they be cankerous or fistulous, with tents rolled therein, or the parts washed or injected

therewith, cleanest them thoroughly from the bottom
and healtheth them up safely. The whole plant of the
greater centaury, as well herb as root, is very available
in all sorts of wounds or ulcers, to dry, solder,
cleanse and heal them, and therefore it is, or should
be, a principal ingredient in all vulnerary drinks and
injections.

Knapweed, which some call dark-bottle,
is good for all those that are bruised by any falls,
beatings, and other casualties: It is very profitable
for them that are bursten, if they drink the decoction
of the herb and root in wine, and apply the same
outwardly to the place. It is singular good also in all
sorts of running and cankerous sores and fistulas,
drying up the moisture, and healing them gently,
without any sharpness or biting; it doth the like also in
the running sores and scabs of the head or other parts.
It is of especial use for the soreness of the throat, the
swellings of the palate and jaws. It is also excellent
for all green wounds, to stay the bleeding, and close
the lips of them together.

All the plantains are singular good wound
herbs to heal fresh and old sores and wounds,
whether inward or outward. The flower of beans and
fenugreek mixed with honey, helpeth felons, boils
and bruises. The roots of white bryony, being bruised
and applied of itself to any place where the bones are
broken, helpeth to draw them forth, as also splinters,
arrowheads and thorns in the flesh; and being applied
with a little wine mixed therewith, it breaketh boils
and helpeth whitlows. The berries of bittersweet, or
woody nightshade, bruised and laid to the finger that

hath a felon thereon, cure it, and so do the leaves
stamped together with crusty bacon.

He that hath sanicle and self-heal to help
himself, needeth neither Physician nor chirurgeon,
so effectual are they in several cases, but especially
in green wounds. Houndstongue is good against
the biting of mad dogs, and is the main ingredient
whereof black salve is made. The inner bark of an
elder tree boiled in vinegar is approved to cure the
itch and take away scabs, and so are decoctions of
scabious and alehoof, or ground-ivy. The fume of the
dried herb, stalk and seeds of henbane burned, quickly
healeth swellings, chilblains, or kibes on the hands or
feet if they be held therein.

Savine, dried into a powder and mixed with
honey, breaketh carbuncles and plague sores; it also
helpeth the King's Evil, being applied unto the place;
being spread upon a piece of leather and applied to
the navel, kills the worms in the belly; it helpeth
scabs, itch, running sores, cankers, tetters and ring
worms.

An hundred more I could reckon up, but let
these suffice for the present.

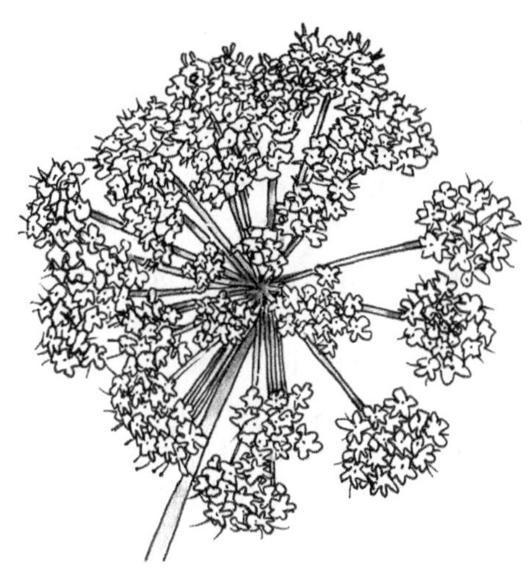

Of Poisonous Plants

Whatsoever is received into the body is either aliment, medicine or poison. Of the two first I have entreated already. I come now to the third; and here I know not whether to call it a civil or rather uncivil use, or abuse, that hath been made of plants in this kind. The form of executing capital offenders in Athens was the taking of the potion of hemlock, which was (for sooth as they pretended) in humanity given to them that their deaths might be with the less pain, and after this manner did Socrates die. The inhabitants of the Isle of Cea, when they were above threescore years old and deemed unfit for the managery of public affairs, did voluntarily take the like potion. Some have used opium (which is the juice of a certain poppy) to the same purpose, but that is more painful because it hath parts of heat mixed.

The juices of garlic, onions and leeks, if taken in any great quantity, are rank poison, although we eat the flesh and all with little or no danger. Lettuce is thought to be poisonous when it is so old as to have milk. Spurge is a kind of poison itself, and so is nightshade, henbane, mandrake and wolf's-bane, of which Master Gerard reports that a gentleman tasting the roots had his tongue and mouth so swollen that it is thought he would have died if he had not met with present help. The yew tree is venomous, both to man and beast. That it is poison to kine will appear by what followeth. Master Wells, minister at Adderbury in Oxfordshire, seeing some boys breaking boughs from the yew tree in the churchyard, thought himself much injured. To prevent the like trespasses, he sent one presently to cut down the tree and to bring it into his backside. This being done, his cows began to feed upon the leaves, and two of them within few hours died. A just reward.

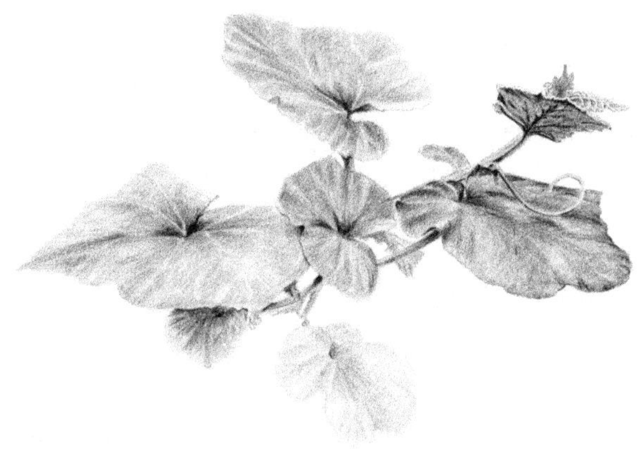

Plants for Making Cloth, Cordage, et cetera

So much for the internal uses of plants, come
we now to the external; and because those which serve
for clothing, are most necessary, we will speak of them
first. There be of plants which are used for garments
these that follow. Hemp and flax grow commonly
in England and are made into cloth by the good
housewives of every country. Cotton is not so well
known, because it grows beyond the seas, as in India,
Arabia, Egypt, *et cetera*. It is an annual plant as hemp,
and unless it be gathered in time, the seeds with the
wool encompassing them fall to the ground. Of this are
made fustions, bombasts, stockings, *et cetera*. In some
countries, for want of the aforesaid materials, they strip
the nettles and make cloth thereof, which must needs
be very course. But finer stuff is made of sericum,
which is a growing silk coming out of the Island Seres,
where it grows upon the leaves of trees, yet some is
made by the silk worms in every country. They make

also cables of the bark of lime trees.

And here I think it will not be impertinent to our present matter to give you to understand that in India there is a tree called the coconut tree, whose leaves serve to cover houses, whose hairy stuff or hards, which is next the outward bark, doth make not only cordage and tackle for ships, but also cloth, cauls and girdles, even for the better sort. There is in the Anatomy School at Oxford, amongst very many curious rarities, a purse made of the bark of a certain outlandish tree.

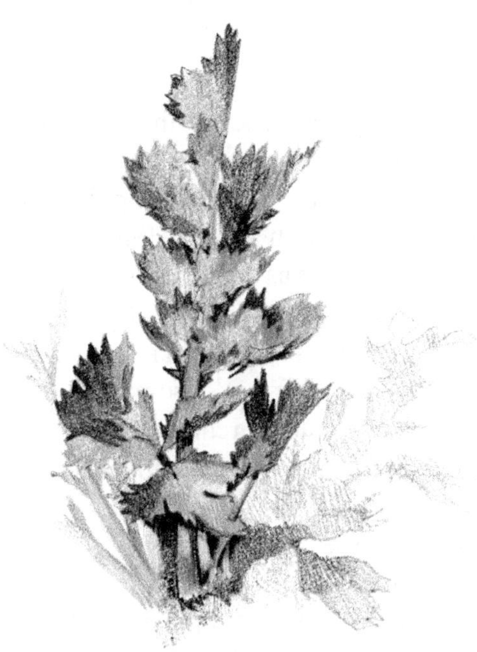

Of the Ornamental Use of Plants Formerly, and What are in Use at This Present

Plants are an ornament to the place where they naturally grow. How bravely are the woods adorned with trees and the meadows with flowers, the gardens with sweet smelling herbs, the walls and house sides with vines and other fruitful trees, insomuch that the psalmist tells the blessed man that his wife shall be as the fruitful vine on the sides of his house, and his Children shall stand like olive branches roundabout his table.

The olive was the emblem of peace, and therefore the door for the entering in of the Oracle in Solomon's Temple were made of olive trees, and so were the lintels and side-posts, it being a time of peace. I know not whether the Athenians did adorn their temples with the branches of the olive also, but surely they had it in so great veneration that they would not suffer a goat to come into the Acropolis where it grew. It is probable enough that the Temple of Minerva, to whom it was sacred, was sometimes dressed with it.

Other heathens also did garnish their temples with laurel, myrtle, oak, *et cetera*. The branches of pines, oaks and apple trees, and also parsley were bestowed upon those that overcame in the Grecian games in token of victory. So the Roman combatants who overcame received by way of reward a garland or coronet of palm tree. The reason why the palm tree, rather than any other tree, should be given in token of victory is rendered by diverse approved authors to be this: because the Palme tree, though you put never so ponderous a heavy weight upon it, yet it will not yield but rather endeavor the more upward. Their generals also in their triumphs heretofore wore a crown of laurel, and when they had raised any siege, they were honored with a crown of grass.

In Ovid's time, the emperor had always standing before his gates an oak tree in the midst of two laurel as an emblem denoting two worthy virtues required in all emperors and princes: first, whereby the enemy might be conquered; secondly, such whereby citizens might be saved. Unto this the poet seemeth to allude speaking of the laurel tree;

Postibus Augustus fidissima cadem Custos
Ante fores status, mediamque tuebere quercum.

It is not very long since the custom of setting up garlands in churches hath been left off with us; and in some places setting up of holly, ivy, rosemary, bays, yew, *et cetera* in Churches at Christmas is still in use. Cypress garlands are of great account at funerals amongst the gentler sort, but rosemary and bays are used by the commons both at funerals and weddings. They are all plants which fade not a good while after they are gathered and used (as I conceive) to intimate unto us that the remembrance of the present solemnity might not die presently, but be kept in mind for many years. Box and ivy last long green, and therefore vintners make their garlands thereof; though perhaps ivy is the rather used because of the antipathy between it and wine. The willow garland is a thing talked of, but I had rather talk of it than wear it.

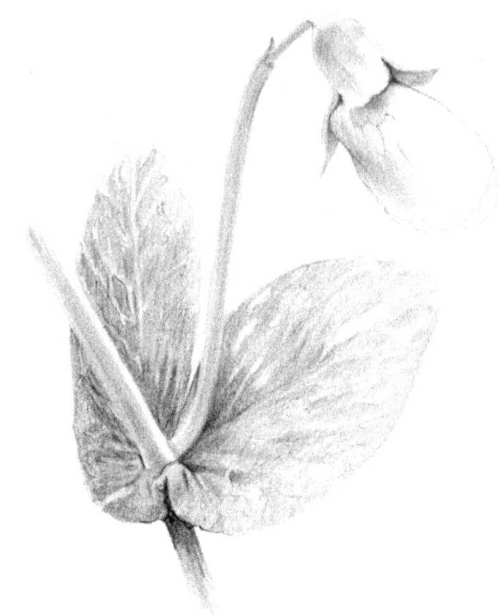

Of Plants Used In and Against Witchcraft

The ointment that witches use is reported to be made of the fat of children digged out of their graves; of the juices of smallage, wolf's-bane and cinquefoil mingled with the meal of fine wheat. But some suppose that the soporiferous medicines are likeliest to do it, which are henbane, hemlock, mandrake, nightshade, tobacco, opium, saffron, poplar leaves, *et cetera*. They take likewise the roots of mandrake, according to some, or as I rather suppose the roots of bryony, which simple folk take for the true mandrake and make thereof an ugly image, by which they intend to exercise their witchcraft.

Many odd wive's fables are written of vervain, which you may read elsewhere, as Master Gerard saith.

Those that are used against witchcraft are

mistletoe, which if one hang about their neck, the witches can have no power of him. The roots of angelica do likewise avail much in the same case, if a man carry them about him, as Fuchsius saith. The common people formerly gathered the leaves of elder upon the last day of April, which to disappoint the charms of witches, they had affixed to their doors and windows. Matthioli saith that herb Paris takes away evil done by witchcraft, and affirms that he knew it to be true by experience. I do not desire any to pin their faiths upon these reports, but only let them know that there are such which they may believe as they please. However, there is no question but very wonderful effects may be wrought by the virtues which are enveloped within the compass of the green mantles, wherewith many plants are adorned.

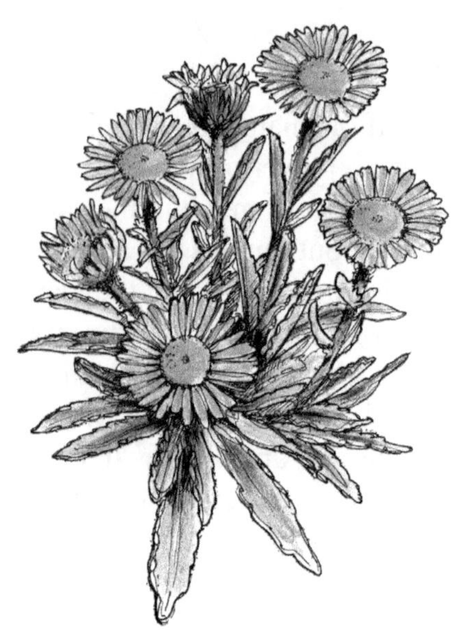

Other Traditions Concerning Plants

It hath been credibly reported to me from several hands that if a man take an elder stick and cut it on both sides so that he preserves the joint, and put in his pocket when he rides a journey, he shall never gall. It is likewise said, that if a handful of arsesmart be put under the saddle upon a tired horseback, it will make him travail fresh and lustily. And if a footman take mugwort and put into his shoes in the morning, he may go forty miles before noon and not be weary. I have read that the lesser moonwort will open locks and pull off the shoes of the horse's feet that pass over it. I have heard that if maids will take wild tansy and lay it to soak in buttermilk for the space of nine days, and wash their faces therewith, it will make them look very fair; that spurge or laurel leaves if be broken off upwards will cause vomiting, if downwards purging; and that the seeds of parsley being eaten cause the falling sickness.

The roots of tarragon and pellitory of Spain, held between the teeth, will make them leave aching. It hath been long received and confirmed by diverse trials that the root of male peony dried, tied to the neck, doth help the incubus, which we call the mare. It is thought that castoreum, musk, rue seed, and agnus seed would do the same.

It hath been observed, that if a woman with child eat quinces much and coriander seed (the nature of both which is to repress and stay vapours that ascend to the brain), it will make the child ingenious. And on the contrary side, if the mother eats much onions or beans, or such vaporous food, it endangereth the child to become lunatic, or of imperfect memory. The leaf of the greater burdock borne or laid on the top of the head, doth draw the matrix upwards; but laid under the soles of the feet, it draweth it downward, which is a notable remedy against the suffocations, falling and displacing of the matrix. I have seen a man lay the leaves aforesaid, to the soles of his feet to cure him of the gout.

All kind of docks have this property, that what flesh or meat is sod therewith, though it be never so old, hard or tough, it will become tender and meet to be eaten. Calamint will recover stinking meat if it be laid amongst it whilst it is raw. The often smelling to basil breedeth a scorpion in the brain. The seed of fleabane strewed between the sheets causeth chastity. Boemus relates that in Darien in America, the women eat an herb when they are great with child that makes them to bring forth without pain. Sowbread is dangerous for women with child, yea so dangerous, that both Dioscorides and Pliny say it will make a woman miscarry if she doe but stride over it, whereby I conceive it may be useful for women that are in travail and cannot easily be delivered. If one that hath eaten Comin do but breathe on a painted face, the colour will vanish away straight. If a man gather vervain the first day of the new moon, before sunrise, and drink the juice thereof, it will make him to avoid lust for seven years. The seeds of docks tied to the left arm of a woman do help barrenness.

I could reckon up many more traditions to such purposes as these concerning plants, but I will not venture to trespass any further upon the reader's patience. Thus have I done with the walls of our cottage, I shall now proceed to the roof.

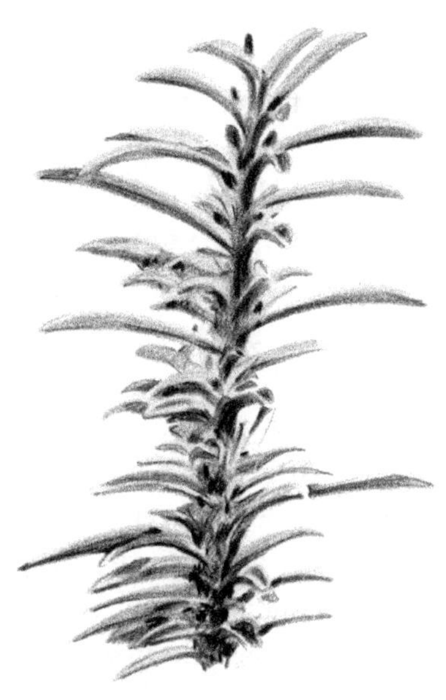

Observations for the Setting of Plants

The diagnostics and uses being thus demonstrated, it is possible that someone may be induced to wish for some directions for the improvement of his garden, to whom especially, but consequently to others, I shall continue my discourse. I am no gardener, nor no gardener's son, yet I hope the gardeners will not be angry with me if I set down a few directions for the more convenient placing of plants in a garden.

It hath been found by woeful experience, that toads do oftentimes lie amongst sage. It would therefore be good to plant one slip of sage, and another of rue, for toads will by no means come nigh unto rue. When you set cabbage plants, make not the hole you set them in down right but sloping so will they more probably come to be cabbages. It is said that if potato roots be set in a pot filled with earth, and then the pot with earth be set likewise within the ground some two or three inches, the roots will grow greater than ordinary. If onions be taken out of the earth and laid a drying twenty days and set again they will be a great deal bigger. The cutting of the leaves of radish or other roots in the beginning of winter before they wither, and covering again the root somewhat high with earth, will preserve the root and make it bigger in the spring following. Rue doth prosper much and become stronger, if it be set by a fig tree, but if it be set by coleworts it will not thrive.

Shade to some plants conduceth to make them large and prosperous more than the sun, as in strawberries and bays, *et cetera*. Therefore, among strawberries sow here and there some borage seed, and you shall find the strawberries under those leaves far more large then their fellows. And bays you must plant to the north, or defend them from the sun by a hedgerow; and when you sow the berries, weed not the borders for the first half year for the weeds give them shade. Scordium likewise delighteth to grow in cool and shadowy places and is found near riversides.

If roots, peas, strawberries and flowers may be accelerated in their coming and ripening (as questionless they may, by making a hot bed with horse-dung and casting earth thereon) there would arise a double profit: the one in the high price that those things bear which come early, the other in the swiftness of their returns. For in some grounds which are strong, you shall have radishes, *et cetera* come in a month, that in other grounds will not come in two, and so make double returns. Or if you water them once in two or three days with water wherein sheep's dung or pigeon's dung hath been steeped, they will come the sooner.

Some plants will not grow near one another, not that there is any antipathy in themselves, but because they draw the same juice and so deceive one another, as the vine and coleworts, a reed and a brake, and hemlock and Rue. Therefore, it would not be amiss to set plants of as contrary juice as you can together.

You must take heed of suffering great trees to grow in your gardens, for besides the droppings of the trees, which most plants will not abide, they so soak and exhaust it that they hurt all plants that grow by them, especially ashes and such trees as spread the roots near the top of the ground. He that desires to be satisfied further that there is no sympathy nor antipathy in plants, let him read the *Historia Naturalis* of the famous and experienced Lord Bacon, who hath treated very judiciously on this subject, of whom I confess I have made use in several places of this treatise, but especially in this chapter.

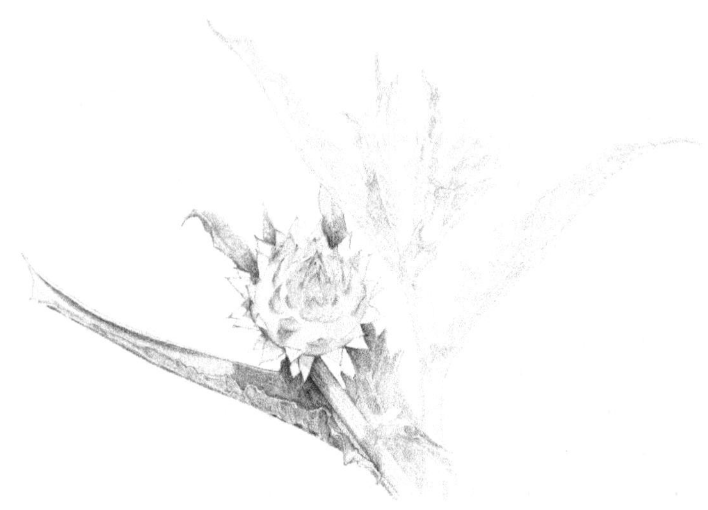

Directions for the Gathering of Plants, and Keeping Them After They are Gathered

And now I have done with the setting of plants, give me leave to speak somewhat of the gathering of them also.

Some of the ancients and diverse modern writers who have professed astrology have noted a sympathy between the sun, moon, some principal stars and certain planets–*for from the influence of those superior bodies are the inferior vegetables, et cetera furnished with their occult qualities*–and so they have denominated some herbs solar and some lunar, and such trifles put into great words. Among them, Master Culpeper (a man now dead, and therefore I shall speak of him as modestly as I can, for were he alive, I should be more plain with him) was a great stickler. And he, indeed, judged all men unfit to be physicians who are not artists in astrology, as if he and some other figure-flinger companions

had been the only physicians in England, whereas
for ought I can gather, either by his books or from
the report of others, he was a man very ignorant in
the form of simples. Many books indeed he hath
tumbled over and transcribed as much out of them as
he thought would serve his turn (though many times
he was therein mistaken) but added very little of his
own [* –saving the scurrility with which he cloaked
his ignorance, and which I am confident can find
agreement with no persons but such as are willing to
be cheated with words].

But to pass by that, how did he think (if
astrologers only can gather herbs) that a man might
cure himself for three pence charge? Did he think
anyone could make a journey to an astrologer
for three pence? Yet I perceive him to be a very
indifferent man, for he saith in his *English Physitian,
enlarged*, where he treateth of gathering simples,
let the planet that governs, *et cetera*, if they can. In
herbs of Saturn, let Saturn be ascendent, let the Moon
apply to them by good aspect, and let her not be in
the house of their enemies; if you cannot well stay
till she apply to them, let her apply to a planet of the
same triplicity. If you cannot waight (sure he or the
printer had not learned to spell) that time neither, let
herbs with a fixed star of their nature, and truly he
might as well have said, if you cannot stay till then,
you may gather them at any time. But I see Master
Culpeper can allow much superstition in himself as
to stargazing, though he rails at it so vehemently in
herbarists of former times for naming plants.

[* Many other learned men have either

defended or favored this opinion; diverse late physicians of other countries (famous for the visible mastery they had over diseases) were not only studious to understand, and did strictly observe the times of collecting their plants for physical uses, but used only those compositions which their apothecaries made up at certain and select hours, and under such positions of planets that suited with, or favored, the nature and quality of the things compounded. And such as diligently applied themselves to know the relation and community between the superiors and inferiors never wanted a good medicine when they stood in need thereof.

I wish that both our physicians and apothecaries would but seriously (without a prejudicated opinion) experiment some few things in this kind. I am confident they would find a manifest difference in their operations and the working of such as are gathered or compounded at uncertain, or contrary, times. But the truth is, the gathering of simples according to particular constellations, and as they ought to be, is a doctrine neither judiciously studied or sufficiently known. If Mr. Culpepper had but in a moderate measure understood this doctrine, or known but the truth of what he has pretended unto, the world had not been abused with such lame and imperfect directions, as he (in his English Physician enlarged) has left unto it. And for ought I can gather either from his books, or learn from the report of others that understood them well, he was a man very ignorant, not only in the forms of simples but in diverse other things he boasts of.

To such therefore as cannot attain the exact knowledge of gathering plants, by an astrological election of fit and suitable times and hours, I shall only prescribe some general rules.]

Now to proceed to the directions.

(1) Though I admit not of Master Culpeper's astrological way of every planet's dominion over plants, yet I conceive that the sun and moon have general influences upon them, the one for heat, the other for moisture; wherein the being of plants consists, and that the full of the moon would be a good time to gather those herbs out of which the juice is to be taken, for then it is most plentiful but for other uses, the leaves newly gathered (if it be not when they are very young or very old) are questionless the best, but at such times, or when they are not at all to be had, we must be glad to make use of the dried ones, which whether dried in the sun or in the shade, so they be neither over nor under dried, it signifieth very little.

(2) Those which you gather for your use in winter, gather a little before they run to seed, for then they be most effectual.

(3) Let them be gathered (as near as you can) from their proper places, which I have directed you to in the first chapter.

(4) For the place you put them in, it matters not, so they lose not their virtue by too much heat, nor corrupt by too much moisture. For flowers, let them be gathered in their prime, dried and laid up as

aforesaid.

(5) For seeds, let them be gathered when they are full ripe and kept not above a year, for afterwards they decay.

(6) What roots you have growing so near you so that you can go to them upon all occasions, trouble not yourself to dry. But if you chance to bring any from afar, hang them somewhat near the fire, otherwise they will rot.

(7) Barks newly gathered are best. Or if the tree whose bark you are to use grow not near, you may take your own time; but they come off easiest in the spring.

(8) For the bark of roots, slit them and take out the pith, and that which remains is called the bark.

(9) If you have occasion to preserve the juice of any herb, pound the herb and strain it, then clarify it by boiling it till no scum rise. When it is cold, fill a glass almost to the neck and fill up the remaining space with oil to keep out the air, or else you may continue boiling it over the fire till it attains unto the consistency of honey, and then it is by physicians called the rob.

[* *Text in brackets from the later 1657 edition of The Art of Simpling.*]

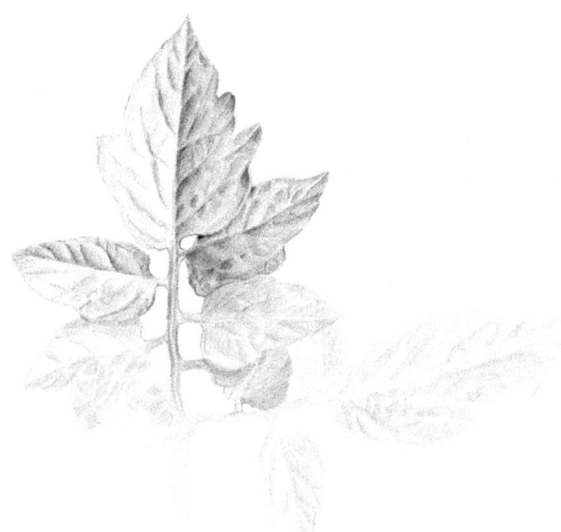

Of the Temperatures or Degrees of Plants

After the gathering of plants, I hold it not amiss to acquaint you with the four prime qualities which are in them, viz., heart, cold, moisture and dryness, and that every one of these have four degrees or orders, which are by several persons diversely defined. But because they are more easily apprehended by the effectual operations which they have to alter a man's body, we will go that way to work.

For seeing that (in this sense) that is temperate, which hath no power eminent to heat, cool, dry or moisten the body of a man, that is accounted the first degree which obscurely and but a little altereth it. The second degree is when the body is manifestly altered, yet without any hurt, offense, or trouble. The third degree is when the body is altered, not only apparently, but also vehemently, not without trouble and offense, yet without corruption. The fourth is that which alters the body most vehemently, and not without very grievous hurt. And every one of these have a triple latitude: intense, remiss, and indifferent.

Temperate Plants and Fruits:

Maidenhair, asparagus, licorice, pine-nuts, figs, raisins, dates, woodruff, bugle, goat's rue, flaxweed, cinquefoil, *et cetera.*

Hot in the First Degree:

Wormwood, marshmallows, borage, bugloss, oxeye, beets, cabbage, chamomile, agrimony, fumitory, wild flax, melilot, comfrey, avens, eyebright, self-heal, chervil, basil, *et cetera*; sweet almonds, chestnuts, cypress nuts, green walnuts, ripe grapes, ripe mulberries, seeds of coriander, flax, gromwell, *et cetera.*

Hot in the Second Degree:

Brooklime, green anise, angelica, parsley, mugwort, betony, ground pine, fenugreek, St. John's-wort, ivy, hops, balm, horehound, rosemary, savory, sage, maudlin, lady's mantle, dill, smallage, marigolds, Carduus benedictus, scurvygrass, alehoof, Alexander, archangel, devil's bit, sanicle, capers, nutmegs, dry figs, dry nuts; the seeds of dill, parsley, rocket, basil, nettle; the roots of parsley, fennel, lovage, mercury, butterbur, hog's fennel, *et cetera.*

Asarabacca, agnus, arum, dry anise, germander, bastard, saffron, centaury, celandine, calamint, fleabane, elecampane, hyssop, bays, marjoram, pennyroyal, rue, savin, bryony, pilewort, bank cress, clary, lavender, feverfew, mint, watercress, hellebore, *et cetera.*

Hot in the Fourth Degree:

Sciatica, cress, spurge, pepper, mustard seed, garlic, leeks, onions, stonecrop, dittander or pepperwort, garden cresses, crowfoot, ros solis, and the root of pellitory of Spain.

Cold in the First Degree:

Orage, mallows, myrtle, pellitory-of-the-wall, sorrel, wood-sorrel, burdock, shepherd's-purse, hawkweed, burnet, coltsfoot, quinces, pears, roses, violets.

Cold in the Second Degree:

Blites, lettuce, duckmeat, endive, hyacinth, plantain, fleawort, nightshade, cucumbers, chickweed, dandelion, fumitory, wild tansy, knotgrass, *et cetera*; oranges, peaches, damsons, *et cetera.*

Cold in the Third Degree:

Purslane, houseleek, everlasting, orpine, *et cetera*; seeds of henbane, hemlock, poppy.

Cold in the Fourth Degree:
Henbane, hemlock, poppies, mandrake, *et cetera.*

Moist in the First Degree:

Bugloss, borage, mallows (their flowers and roots), pellitory, marigolds, basil, the roots of satyrion, *et cetera.*

Moist in the Second Degree:

Violets, waterlily, orage, blites, lettuce, duckmeat, purslane, peaches, damsons, grapes, chickweed, *et cetera.*

Dry in the First Degree:

Agrimony, chamomile, eyebright, self-heal, fennel, myrtle, melilot, chestnuts, beans, barley, *et cetera.*

Dry in the Second Degree:

Pimpernel, shepherd's-purse, wormwood, vervain, mugwort, betony, horsetail, mint, scabious, bugle, Carduus benedictus.

Dry in the Third Degree:

Southernwood, fern, yarrow, cinquefoil, angelica, pilewort, marjoram, rue, savory, tansy, thyme, hellebore.

Dry in the Fourth Degree:

Garden cresses, wild rue, leeks, onions, garlic, crowfoot.

But now methinks I hear some of the common people say, "To what purpose do you tell us of these degrees? We are little wiser than we were before as to the curing of a disease." Observe therefore that all diseases are cured by their contraries, so that if the disease you would cure be hot, as a fever, you must not use wormwood, mint, or anything that is hot, but that which is cooling, as sorrel, endive, violet and strawberry leaves, *et cetera*. In such diseases as proceed of cold, as in cold rhumes, hot things are to be used, as aniseed, fennel seed, betony, rosemary, chamomile flowers, *et cetera*.

But for those that are in health, and their bodies need no alteration, the most temperate are the best, as coming nearest to a man's constitution. But in case you take anything that exceedeth in heat or cold, correct it with its contrary, as Cucumbers are cold and moist, and therefore they are corrected with pepper, which is hot and dry. In gathering sallets, if you put tarragon or garden cresses amongst lettuce, the heat of the one will qualify the coldness of the other and so render them less alterative to a man's body.

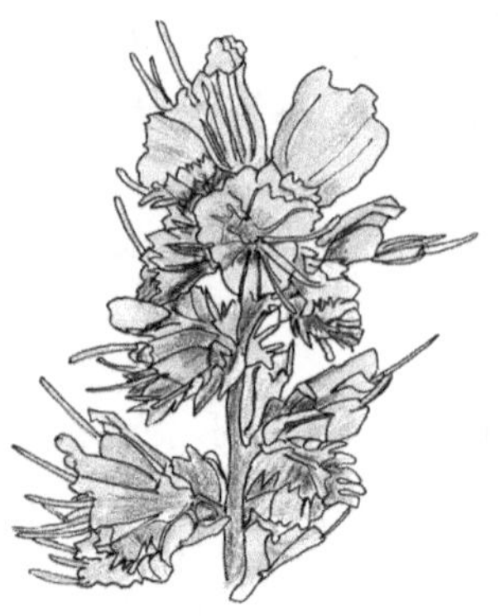

Of the Signatures of Plants

Though sin and Satan have plunged mankind into an ocean of infirmities (for before the Fall, Mankind was not subject to diseases), yet the mercy of God, which is over all his works, maketh grass to grow upon the mountains and herbs for the use of men, and hath not only stamped upon them (as upon every man) a distinct form, but also given them particular signatures whereby a man may read, even in legible characters, the use of them.

That plant that is called adder's-tongue, because the stalk of it represents one, is a sovereign wound herb to cure the biting of an adder, or any other venomous creature. Viper's bugloss hath its stalks all to be speckled like a snake or viper, and is a most singular remedy against poisons and the stinging of scorpions, and other venomous beasts. If a man do but rub his hands with the leaves or roots of dragons, no serpent will endure to come near him, as Dioscorides writeth.

There be some satyrions which are just like the stones of a man. One of them is full and plump and sinks if it be put in water, and that provokes lust; the other swims and is lank and shriveled, and that mortifies it; so that there is a remedy for him in both cases.

Heart trefoil is so called, not only because the leaf is triangular like the heart of a man, but also because each leaf contains the perfect icon of an heart, and that in its proper colour, viz. a flesh colour. It defendeth the heart against the noisome vapor of the spleen. Another trefoil hath a white spot in the leaf like a pearl, and is of singular virtue against the pearl or pin and web in the eye. And there is another trefoil called purplewort, which is an excellent remedy against the purples.

Houndstongue hath a form not much different from its name; it will tie the tongues of hounds so that they shall not bark at you, if it be laid under the bottoms of one's feet, as Miraldus written. If the root of Solomon's-seal be like a seal (as some say it is), it is a good signature for it seals up wounds after a wonderful manner. There are some that say that the leaves of elder do mollify and discuss scirrhous tumors by signature because it groweth in dark and shadowy places. But walnuts bear the whole signature of the head: the outward most green bark answerable to the thick skin wherewith the head is covered, and a salt made of it is singularly good for wounds in that part; as the kernel is good for the brains, which it resembles, being environed with a shell, which imitates the skull, and then it is wrapped up again in a silken covering somewhat representing the pia mater.

The decoction of quinces which are a downy

and hairy fruit is accounted good for the fetching
again hair that hath fallen by the French pox. The lye
wherein maidenhair is sodden, or infused, is good
to bathe the head and make the hair come thicker in
those places which are more thin and bare. The leaves
of St. John's-wort, seem to be pricked or pinked very
thick with little holes like the pores of a man's skin.
It is a sovereign remedy for any cut in the skin and
useful also for the opening of the pores of the body
when they are obstructed.

The flower of arum, or cuckoo-pint, hath the
evident resemblance of the genital parts upon it and
is a most powerful incentive to lust. The poisonous
gum thistle called Euphorbia doth bear evident tokens
of the hot and inflaming sharpness wherewith it is
endued. And I know not why Sagittaria, or arrowhead,
should not be good for wounds made with the head
of an arrow, and kidney beans for diseases of the
kidneys, though I confess I have not read to that
purpose in any author. But pimpernel, and generally
all such plants as are speckled with spots like the
skins of vipers of other venomous creatures, are
known to be good against the stings or bitings of them
and are powerful antidotes against poison.

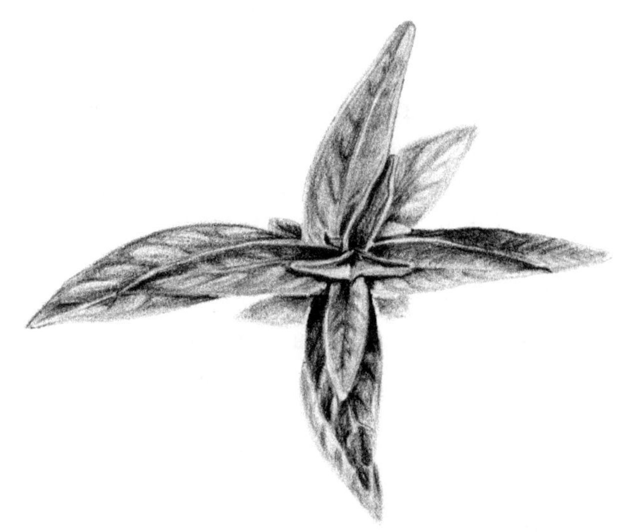

Of Plants That Have No Signatures

But because all plants have not their
signatures, we are not rashly to conclude that they
are therefore unfit for medicinal uses, there being
no necessity that all should be thus signed though
some be, for then the rarity of it, which is the delight,
would be taken away by too much harping upon one
string. Therefore, being thus initiated and entered
into the useful knowledge of plants by signatures, we
must cast ourselves with great courage and industry
(as some before us have done) upon attempting the
virtues of them which are yet undiscovered. For man
was not brought into the world to live like an idle
loiterer or truant, but to exercise his mind in those
things which are therefore in some measure obscure
and intricate, yet not so much as otherwise they would
have been, it being easier to add than invent at first.

And now I shall instance in a few things
commonly accounted useless and unprofitable, as in

stinking weeds and poisonous plants, how that they
were not created in vain but have their uses. They
would not be without their use if they were good for
nothing else but to exercise the industry of man to
weed them out, who had he nothing to struggle with,
the fire of his spirit would be half extinguished in
the flesh. But further, why may not poisonous plants
draw to them all the malign juice and nourishment
that the other may be more pure and refined, as well
as toads and other poisonous serpents lick the venom
from the earth, or that the gall of man should drain
his body of superfluous choler? Certain it is that
many herbs, which the rude and ignorant call weeds,
are the ingredients of very sovereign medicines.
Winter wolf's-bane, which otherwise is rank poison,
is reported to prevail mightily against the bitings of
scorpions and vipers. So have I seen some people
when they have burned their fingers to go and burn
them again to fetch out the fire. And why may not
one poison fetch out another, as well as fire fetch out
fire? And that nightshade, which carries death in its
very name, prevents death by procuring sleep if it be
rightly applied in a fever. It is supposed that hemlock
and henbane may do the same in desperate diseases
which require desperate cures. Hellebore is a simple
which is dangerous to be given to delicate bodies
without great correction, yet it may be safely given
to country people, who have tough bodies. So that
the constitution of the party receiving, as well as the
quality of the thing to be received, is to be considered,
for that which is one man's meat, is another man's
poison. Mallows, pellitory and mercury are reckoned

weeds by the vulgar, and yet they are three of the five emollient herbs, which are used in every glister.

Thus have those plants which have no signatures very great use in physick, and so have they, questionless, which are not yet discovered, though they be left by providence for the enquiry of succeeding ages. For should all things be known at once, posterity would have nothing left wherewith to gratify themselves in their own discoveries, which is a great encouragement to active and quick wits, to make them enquire into those things which are hid from the eyes of those which are so dull and stupid that they relish all objects alike; though they have the use of eyes as well as other folks, yet they see not, or at least take no notice of the outward forms of things, much less the inward power, and secret virtue wherewith every plant is endued.

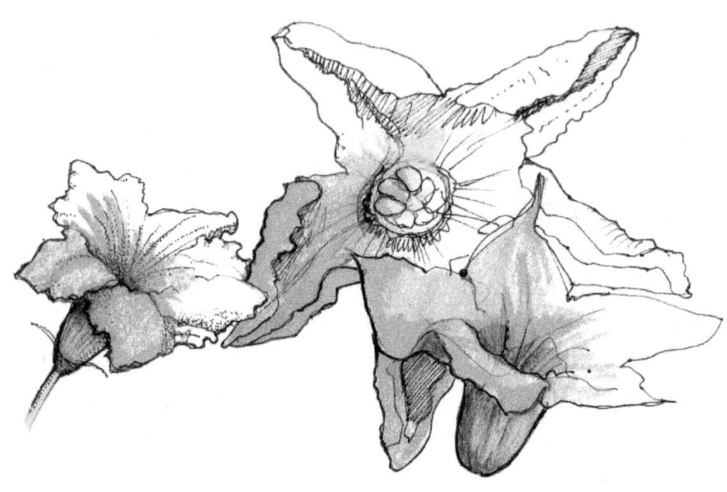

What Plants are Profitable for Every Part

It will not (as I suppose) be altogether unreasonable or impertinent before I conclude to set down somewhat more particularly what plants do most properly belong to every part. For you must know that those which are good for one part may be hurtful to another; yet the same plant, which in some diseases is profitable, is in other some hurtful, unless it be prepared and corrected by a skillful hand, there being in them besides their first quality, some second and secret ones which may very much annoy the body. And some plants though they are good for some parts, yet are altogether destructive to others, as I shall show in the next chapter. In this I shall speak only of those which maintain the welfare of every part and cure, it being distempered. And because the head is the principal part of man, I shall begin with that and so descend downwards. And for as much as there seldom happens a single distemper, but it hath some other concomitant, as Heat is wont to be joined with dryness, and cold with moisture, I shall therefore comprehend those that heat and dry under one title, and those that cool and moisten under another.

Those That Heat and Dry the Head:

Such as are well scented yet not over-strong, for strong scents cause the headache by filling it with vapor: betony, marjoram, sage, hyssop, balm, rosemary, which strengthens the senses and memory and is good for the palsy; the leaves and berries of bays, savory, rue, calamint, lavender, oregano, cowslips, lily-of-the-valley, cassidony (which helpeth the nerves and therefore ought to be used in all remedies that belong to them), chamomile, basil, clove gillyflowers, melilote, peony; the seeds of lovage and fennel; the root of the flower-de-luce; the flowers of the lime tree, juniper berries, coriander, mistletoe, which cureth the falling sickness, rhubarb, *et cetera.*

Those That Cool and Moisten the Head:

Roses, which strengthen the brain; violets, which provoke sleep and allay the acrimony of choler; flowers of waterlily; the leaves and seeds of lettuce, purslane, poppy seed, wood sorrel. To which may be added those which are more moist and fitter for melancholy diseases, viz. borage, bugloss, sweet smelling apples and sweet almonds, all which may be applied outwardly also to cool the head. And besides

these nightshade, everlasting, violet leaves, the leaves
of willows, but especially of roses and whatsoever
is made of them, for they refresh the brain with their
sweet odour and drive away vapors from thence.

Those That are Good for the Eyes:

Fennel, eyebright, rue, vervain, celandine,
marjoram, betony, elecampane, rhubarb, the roots of
valerian, the seeds of clary (but especially of the wild
sort, which is called Oculus Christi) one of which
being put into each eye cleanseth them and purgeth
them exceedingly from waterish humors, redness and
inflammation, and diverse other maladies, if not all
that happen unto the eyes, and taketh away the pain
and smarting of.

Those That are Good for the Ears:

If the distemper proceed of cold, rue, bays,
alecost, gith, bitter almonds, onions, white hellebore
with honey, hyssop, the juice of savory heated
with a little oil of roses and dropped into the ears,
easeth them of the noise and singing in them, and
of deafness also, and so doth the juice of sweet
marjoram. If the distemper proceed of heat, roses,
mallows, violets, willow leaves, lettuce, water lilies,
the oil of apricots and peaches, *et cetera.*

Those That Heat and Dry the Breast and Lungs:

Hyssop, scabious, which also openeth

imposthumes in the breast; maidenhair, coltsfoot,
which, taken in a pipe and swallowed down, breaketh
imposthumes; horehound, calamint, betony, fluellen,
Carduus benedictus, licorice, the roots of elecampane,
and flower-de-luce, round birthwort, which prevaileth
much against inward imposthumes and thick phlegm;
nettle seeds, fennel seeds, figs, raisins, almonds,
the roots of arum, dragons, burnet, linseed, nettles,
rhubarb.

Those That Cool and Moisten the Breast and Lungs:
Violets, mallows, the seeds of white poppy and
fleabane, broth made of French barley, *et cetera*,
which allay the hot and sharp humors, moisten the
lungs being dry, and make smooth the rough passages.

Those That Heat the Heart:

Rosemary, balm, basil, Carduus benedictus,
water germander, fluellin, the barks and seeds of
citrons, clove gillyflowers, angelica roots, and those
of elecampane, marigold flowers, mace, nutmegs,
cinnamon, cloves, saffron, southernwood, goat's rue,
woodruff.

Those That Cool the Heart and Resist Dryness:

Roses, violets, sorrel, bugloss, waterlily,
plantain, the juice of lemons, oranges and
pomegranates, cherries, sweet smelling apples,
raspberries, strawberry leaves.

Those That Heat and Dry the Stomach:

Mint, wormwood, fennel, rosemary, sage, the leaves of bays, the berries of bays and juniper, the seeds of caraway, anise, cumin, smallage, avens, balm, parsley, thyme, rhubarb, *et cetera*.

Those That Cool the Stomach:

Sorrel, sheep's sorrel, purslane, lettuce, plantain, endive, sowthistles, chicory, roses, violets, peaches, quinces, melons, cucumbers, pears, garden corinths, barberries, the juice of lemons, medlars, strawberries, mulberries, *et cetera*.

Those That Heat the Liver:

Agrimony, wormwood, maidenhair, sage, dodder, asarabacca, liverwort, spike, maudlin, fennel, Alexanders, parsley, asparagus, bitter almonds, elecampane, the seeds of anise, caraway, cumin, *et cetera*.

Those That Cool the Liver:

Endive, succory, clary, dandelion, purslane, lettuce, roses, violets, water lilies, sorrel, strawberries, the seeds of melons, gourds, cucumbers, citrulls, endive, lettuce, clary, parsley, French barley, *et cetera*.

Those That Heat the Spleen:

Spleenwort, or miltwaste, wormwood, dodder, fumitory, hops, rue, calamint, Alexanders, fluellen, germander, ground pine, balm, cresses, scurvygrass, horehound, broom, elder, asarabacca, the roots of polypody, elecampane, felwort, fern, fennel, parsley, agnus, tamarisk, capers, birthwort, madder, bitter almonds, *et cetera*.

Those That Cool the Spleen:

Succory, endive, purslane, lettuce willow leaves, sorrel, dandelion, barberies, strawberries, cherries, *et cetera*.

Those That Warm the Reins and Bladder:

Maidenhair, rue, saxifrage, betony, privet, fennel, rocket, mugwort, horseradish, calamint, sea holly, asparagus, butcher's-broom, burnet, licorice, Alexanders, parsley, nettles, wild carrots, dropwort, madder, juniper berries, chamomile flowers, chervil, almonds, the kernels of peaches, cherries, *et cetera*.

Those That Cool the Reins and Bladder:

Knotgrass, mallows, yarrow, moneywort, plantain, endive, succory, lettuce, purslane, water lilies, houseleek, pellitory, the seeds of poppy, fleabane, pompions, *et cetera*.

Those That Heat the Womb:

Mugwort, motherwort, betony, dittany, oregano, pennyroyal, calamint, marjoram, sage, thyme, balm, savory, rue, rosemary, bay leaves, chamomile flowers, the seeds of cumin, anise, fennel, wild carrot, parsley, Alexanders, the roots of birthwort, madder, sea holly, fennel, Alexanders, asparagus, burnet, angelica, valerian, masterwort, *et cetera.*

Those That Cool the Womb:
Water lilies, violets, roses, quinces and their syrup, purslane, lettuce, clary, wild tansy, orache, burdocks, willow-weed, myrtle leaves, moneywort, sowthistles, endive, succory, *et cetera.*

Those That Heat the Joints:

Cowslips, sciatica, cresses, marjoram, betony, hot arsesmart, sage, agrimony, chamomile, St. John's-wort, melilots, mugwort, rosemary, bay leaves, lavender, *et cetera.*

Those That Cool the Joints:

Plantain, willow leaves, vine leaves, lettuce, henbane, nightshade, houseleek, water betony, the inner bark of elm, *et cetera.*

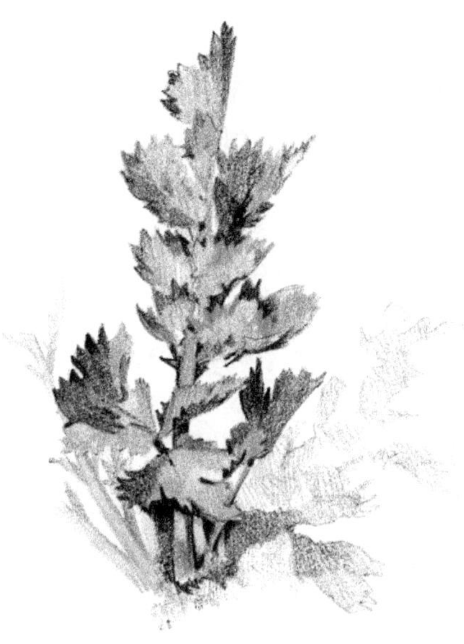

What Plants are Destructive to Every Part

As there be plants profitable for every part, so there be some, though not so many, which are somewhat destructive to some particular parts if not corrected with the mixture of some other ingredients. For though an herb be good for the stomach, it may be naught for the head, and that which is good for the head, may be naught for the stomach. And therefore, I think it will be worthwhile to set them down too, according to my promise made in the foregoing chapter.

Those That are Offensive to the Head:

The seeds of agnus, ivy taken inwardly, camel's hay, the seed of meadowsweet, hemp seed, rocket, horseradish, garlic, onions, leeks,

cedar berries, bitter vetch, the juice of wormwood,
acorns, black olives, the fruit of the strawberry
tree, frankincense taken immoderately, the fruit of
the mastic tree, saffron, hog's fennel, sowbread,
mandrake, hemlock, *et cetera*.

Those That are Offensive to the Eyes:

Dill, lentils, hemp, lettuce, beans, radish,
cabbage, mustard seed, onions, leeks, garlic, *et cetera*.

Those That are Offensive to the Heart:

Spurge, broom.

Those That are Offensive to the Stomach:

Hyssop, Soldanella, flower-de-luce, alder,
spurge, broom, fern, mushrooms, beets, distaff thistle.

Those That are Offensive to Conception:

Spleenwort, colloquintida, wild cucumbers,
scammony, savine, hemp seed, the seeds of agnus.

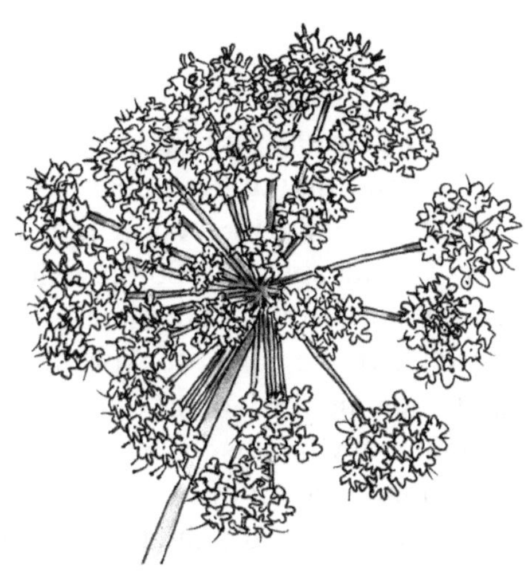

Of Such Plants as Have Operation Upon the Bodies of Brute Beasts

Though the bodies of men be more tender than any other creatures, fuller of diseases, and easier to be wrought upon, and so the greatest number of plants is applicable to them, yet brute beasts also have some share in the physical use of plants as well as they. For a toad being over-charged with the poison of the spider, as is ordinarily believed, hath recourse to the plantain leaf which cures him. The weasel, when she is to encounter the serpent, arms herself with eating of rue. The dog, when he is sick at the stomach, knows the grass that will cure him, eats of it, falls to his vomit, and is well. When the cat is sick, she goes to the nep or catmint, of which there is this old rhyme:

If you set it, the cats will eat it.
If you sow it, the cats can't know it.

If the ass be oppressed with melancholy,
he eats of the herb *Asplenium,* or miltwaste, and so
eases himself of the swelling of the spleen. (Vitruvius
saith that the swine in Candy, by feeding thereon,
were found to be without spleens.) So the wild goats,
being shot with darts or arrows, cure themselves
with dittany, which hath the power to work them out
of the body and to heal up the wound. The swallow
makes use of celandine, which is therefore called
Chelidonium; the linnet and goldfinch of eyebright,
for the repairing of their own and their young one's
sight.

And here, though I am no leech, yet I shall set
down such plants as I have seen and read are used by
leeches, and the manner of applying them to cattle,
and such unusual accidents as happened to them by
their operation. The leaves of black bryony, bruised
with wine and laid upon the forenecks of oxen that are
galled with the yoke, helpeth them. When a cow hath
newly calved, they give her unthreshed rye out of the
barn to make her clean, as they call it. It the calf be
dead in the cow's belly, they give her savine to make
her cast it. When a cow is troubled with the tail evil,
they make an incision towards the lower end of the
tail where the evil is and put therein rue, pepper and
salt, which will cure them. And if hogs or other cattle
be subject to the murrain, it is usual with them, and
almost with every husbandman, to cut an hole in the
ear or dewlap, and put therein a piece of the root of
bear's foot, which some call pegging, some steering,
and therefore the plant is by some called setterwort.

Hay sodden in water till it be tender, and applied hot the chaps of beasts which are chap-fallen, through too much abstinence, either by long standing in the pound or stable without meat, is a present remedy. Ground ivy stamped and mixed with a little ale and honey and strained, taketh away the pin and web, or any grief out of the eyes of horses or cows, or other beast, being squirted into the same with a syringe.

It is reported that if one cast *Lysimachia,* or loosestrife, between two oxen when they are fighting, they will part presently, and being tied about their necks it will keep them from fighting. Cocks having eaten garlic are most stout to fight, and so are horses. A serpent doth so hate the ash tree, that she will not come nigh the shadow of it, but she delights in fennel very much, which she eats to clear her eyesight. If you are troubled with moles in your gardens or other grounds, put garlic, leeks or onions in their passages, and they will leap out of the ground presently. Adder's-tongue, wrapped in virgin-wax and put into the left era of any horse, will make him fall down as if he were dead, and when it is taken out again, he becomes more lively than he was before.

If asses chance to feed much upon hemlock, they will fall so fast asleep that they will seem to be dead, in so much that some thinking them to be dead indeed have flayed off their skins; yet after the hemlock had done operating, they have stirred and wakened out of their sleep, to the grief and amazement of the owners, and to the laughter of others. If a horse cannot piss without pain, take an

elder bough full of leaves and strike him gently
therewith, and cover his head, neck and body with
the same leaves and it will help him much. Wood
nightshade, or bittersweet, being hung about the neck
of cattle that have the staggers helpeth them.

The roots of gentian, or the juice of them,
or the decoction of the herb or root, being given to
cattle to drink, freeth them from the botts and worms,
and many other diseases. As also when they begin to
swell being poisoned by any venomous worm or tick,
which they often lick up with the grass, as also when
such worms, or other hurtful vermin, have bitten kine
by the udders or other tender places, which presently
thereupon swell and put them to so great pain that it
makes them forsake their meat, do but take the leaves
of gentian and stroke the bitten place with the juice of
them, and they by two or three times are helped and
cured.

He that desires further information in cures
of this nature, let him read the works of Gervase
Markham, who hath done very well upon this subject.

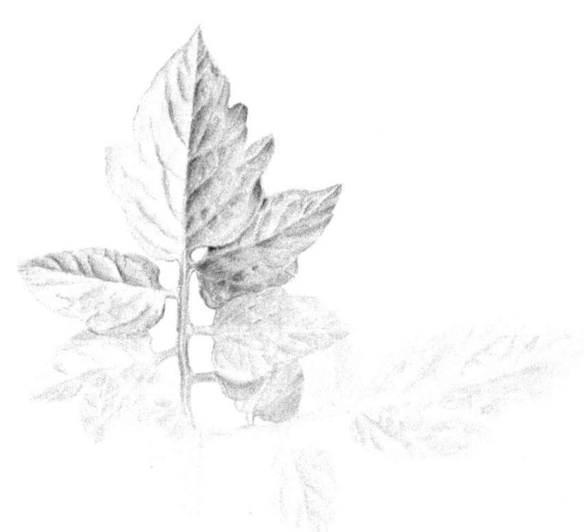

Of the Speculative and Pleasant Use of a Garden

To leave off the properties of simples, we come now to the conveniences of a garden, which are manifold in respect of speculation, by which I mean mere walking, or at most but gathering such things as please them, which I count no labour, for that I extend to oppose as the practical use. That there is no place more pleasant, may appear from God himself, who after he had made man, planted the Garden of Eden and put him therein that he might contemplate the many wonderful ornaments wherewith omnipotence had bedecked his Mother Earth. It was not so much for Adam's recreation, who at that time was not acquainted with weariness, as it was for his instruction, but to us it will serve for both. There is not a plant which grows but carries along with it the legible characters of a deity, according to the verse:

Presentemque refert quoelibet herba Deum.
As for recreation, if a man be wearied with

over-much study (for study is a weariness to the flesh as Solomon by experience can tell you), there is no better place in the world to recreate himself than a garden, there being no sense but may be delighted therein. If his sight be obfuscated and dull, as it may easily be with continual poring, there is no better way to relieve it than to view the pleasant greenness of herbs, which is the way that painters use, when they have almost spent their sight by their most earnest contemplation of brighter objects.

Neither do they only feed the eyes, but comfort the wearied brain with fragrant smells, which yield a certain kind of nourishment, as will appear by the following stories. My Lord Bacon in his Historia Naturalis reporteth, that he knew a gentleman that would fast sometimes four or five days without any manner of sustenance. In which time, he would have lying by him a wisp of herbs, to which he would smell now and then, having in it, garlic, onions and other esculents of strong scent. Doctor Hackwill in his Apology for the worlds not decaying, tells a story of a German gentlewoman who lived fourteen years without receiving any nourishment down her throat, but only walked frequently in a spacious garden full of odoriferous herbs and flowers. That this is possible is further apparent by the story of Democritus, who when he lay a dying, heard his nurse-keeper complain that she should be kept from being at a feast and solemnity (which she much desired to see) because there would be a corpse in the house; whereupon he caused loaves of new bread to be sent for, and opened them, and so kept himself alive with the odour of them till the feast was past.

The ears also (which are called the Daughters of Music because they delight therein) have their recreation by the pleasant noise of the warbling notes, which the chanting birds accent forth from amongst the murmuring leaves. As for the taste, they serve it so exceedingly, that whether it be affected with sweet, sour or bitter things, they even prostitute themselves. And for the feeling likewise, they entertain it with as great variety as can be imagined, there being some plants as soft as silk, and some as prickly as an hedgehog. So, that there is no outward sense which can want satisfaction in this cornucopia.

And if the outward senses be so delighted, the inward will be so too, it being as it were, the School of Memory and Fancy. Hereupon it was that the ancient poets did so much extoll the gardens of Alcinous and the Hesperides. The grove of Mars was not unknown to Juvenal, neither were there any poets which had not recesses into those sacred places. The first institutor of them at Athens was Epicurus, in which he had a school where he taught, one that knew as much what belonged to pleasure as any man. Seneca the philosopher was likewise a great admirer of them, and is said to have expended vast sums of money this way.

A house though otherwise beautiful, yet if it hath no garden belonging to it, is more like a prison than a house.

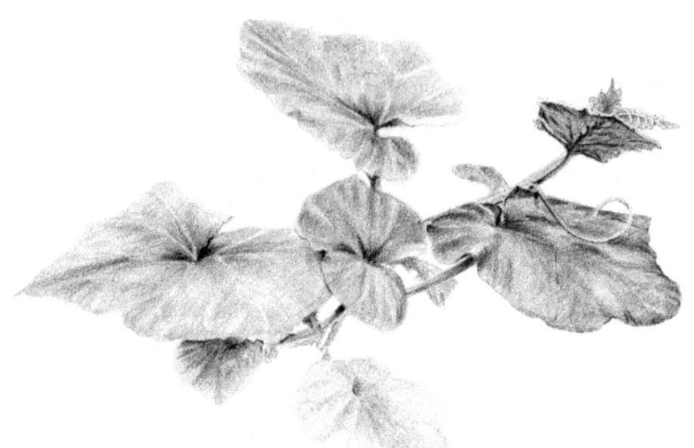

Of the Practical and Profitable Use of a Garden

The pleasure of a garden being thus demonstrated, I shall conclude all with the profit thereof, which is likewise manifold. First, for household occasions, for there is not a day passeth over our heads but we have need of one thing or other that groweth within their circumference. We cannot make so much as a little good pottage without herbs, which give an admirable relish, and make them wholesome for our bodies. In a garden there be turnips and carrots, which serve for sauce, and if meat be wanting, for that too. Neither doth it afford us aliment only, but physick, (no herbs being without their physical use, as I have said before, especially if it be well furnished with simples).

But besides this inestimable profit, there is another not much inferior to it, and that is the wholesome exercise a man may use in it. Dr. Pinck, late warden of New College in Oxon, whereof I was once a member (whose memory I very much honor), was a very learned man and well versed in physick; and truly he would rise very betimes in the morning, even in his later days when he was almost fourscore

years old, and going into his garden he would take
a mattock or spade, digging there an hour or two,
which he found very advantageous to his health. A
man worthy to be imitated, not only in this, but also
in many other things, especially in his charitable
provisions for bringing up of poor children. And if
gentlemen who have little else to do would be ruled
by me, I would advise them to spend their spare time
in their gardens, either in digging, setting, weeding,
or the like, then which there is no better way in the
world to preserve health.

If a man want an appetite to his victuals, the
smell of the earth new turned up by digging with
a spade will procure it, and if he be inclined to a
consumption it will recover him. Gentlewomen, if the
ground be not too wet, may do themselves much good
by kneeling upon a cushion and weeding. And thus
both sexes might divert themselves from idleness,
and evil company, which oftentimes prove the ruin of
many ingenious people.

But perhaps they may think it a disparagement
to the condition they are in; truly none at all, if it were
but put in practice. For we see that those fashions
which sometimes seem ridiculous, if once taken up
by the gentry, cease to be so. And if you shall require
another precedent besides that before mentioned, I
shall present unto you that of the wise and mighty
Emperor Diocletian, who after he had reigned
eighteen years, left for a season the whole government
of the empire, and forsaking the court, betook himself
to a mean house with a garden adjoining, wherein
with his own hands, he both sowed, set, and weeded

the herbs of his garden; which kind of life so pleased
him, that he was hardly entreated to resume the
government of the empire.

    By this time I hope you will think it no
dishonor to follow the steps of our grandsire Adam,
who is commonly pictured with a spade in his
hand, to march through the quarters of your garden
with the like instrument, and there to rectify all the
disorders thereof, to procure, as much as in you
lies, the recovery of the languishing art of simpling,
which did it but appear in lively colours, I am almost
persuaded, it would so affect you, that you would
be much taken with it. There is no better way to
understand the benefit of it, than by being acquainted
with herbals, the herbarists, and by putting this
gentle and ingenious exercise in practice, that so this
part of knowledge, as well as others, may receive
that esteem and advancement that is due to it, to the
banishment of barbarism and ignorance, which begin
again to prevail against it. So that this Art, with the
rest, being improved, may bring forth much glory to
God, much honour to the nation, much pleasure and
profit to those that delight in it, and much comfort to
those which have need of physick. To which end, the
Right Honourable Earle of Danby erected the physick
garden in Oxford, a place worth the seeing.

    And thus you have the unpolished structure of
simpling:

Omne tulit punctum qui miscuit utile dulci.

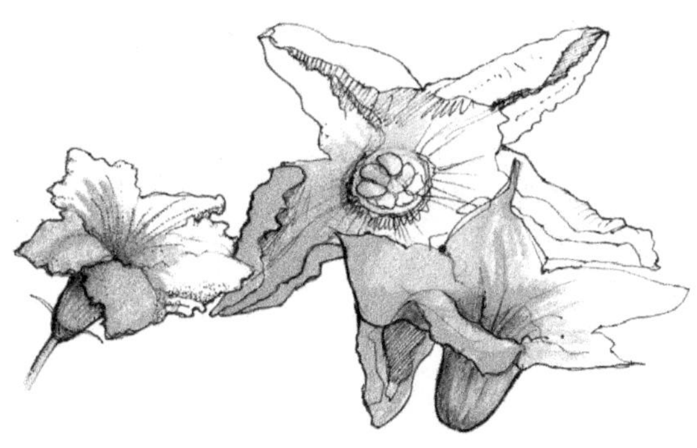

About the Author

William Coles, son of Joh. Cole, a bachelor of divinity and school master at Adderbury grammar school, was born in 1626 in Adderbury, Oxfordshire and educated there at the Boys School. At the age of sixteen, he entered New College at University of Oxford and soon after was made a portionist, commonly called post master, of Merton College by his mother's brother, John French, one of the senior fellows of that house and public registrar of the university.

While a student, Coles also became qualified as a public notary so that he could stand in for his uncle as registrar. Coles took his bachelor of arts degree in 1650, then left Oxford for London and lived for several years at Putney where he became a well-known simpler. Upon the king's restoration in 1660, he was made secretary to Dr. Brian Duppa, bishop of Winchester, in whose service he died in 1662. His published works are the following: The Art of Simpling. London, 1656.; Perspicillum Microcosmologium. London, 1656.; Adam in Eden: or, Nature's Paradise. London, 1657.

from Athenae Oxonienses, v. 3, by Anthony A. Wood. (1817 edition)